Television and Health Responsibility in an Age of Individualism

Television and Health Responsibility in an Age of Individualism

Katherine A. Foss

LEXINGTON BOOKS
Lanham • Boulder • New York • London

Published by Lexington Books
An imprint of The Rowman & Littlefield Publishing Group, Inc.
4501 Forbes Boulevard, Suite 200, Lanham, Maryland 20706
www.rowman.com

16 Carlisle Street, London W1D 3BT, United Kingdom

British Library Cataloguing in Publication Information Available

Library of Congress Cataloging-in-Publication Data

Foss, Katherine A., 1980- , author.
Television and health responsibility in an age of individualism / Katherine A. Foss.
p. cm.
Includes bibliographical references and index.
Television and health responsibility in an age of individualism / Katherine A. Foss.
1. Title.
[DNLM: 1. Physicians. 2. Physician's Role. 3. Physician-Patient Relations. 4. Television. W 62]
610.69'6—dc23
2014029654

Printed in the United States of America

Contents

Acknowledgments

I began this project in 2006 as my dissertation research. Eight years (a Ph.D., tenure, and two kids) later, it has evolved into this book. I am truly thankful to Alison Pavan and Lexington Press for the opportunity to publish this work.

I am grateful to so many people for helping me through this process. My wonderful dissertation advisers, Hazel Dicken-Garcia and Kathy Forde, never failed to answer questions or quickly provide feedback. From them, I learned so much about writing, work ethic, and how to help my own students. Even now, long after the defense, they continue to answer my questions. I also appreciate the wisdom and support of the rest of the faculty and staff at the University of Minnesota. My education solidly prepared me for the tenure track.

This book would not have been possible without the resources and support I have received at Middle Tennessee State University. Funding for conferences and summer research greatly aided the development of this book. I would like to thank the Director of the School of Journalism, Dwight Brooks, and Ken Paulson, the Dean of College of Mass Communication, as well as my fabulous colleagues and our administrative staff. The abundant hallway exchanges and more formal research discussions have kept me thinking. My sincere gratitude goes toward my mentor and friend, Jane Marcellus, for guiding me as a new faculty member and through the publishing process.

It is sometimes difficult to stay the course with a long-term project. My writing group helped me to set and keep deadlines, read drafts of my proposals, and pushed me to finish. A special thanks to Tanya Peres Lemons, who makes writing sessions fun, yet fruitful, and always offers sound and encouraging advice. I also give a nod to the many others that have contributed to this work—members of the Cultural and Critical Studies and other divisions of AEJMC, along with reviewers, discussants, and other folks that have shaped me as a scholar.

On a personal note, I would like to thank my family and friends for their support. Thank you to my parents for letting me watch *Emergency!* at a young age and for sharing their experiences in the medical field. I am indebted to my dear sister, Kristi, for listening to my daily ramblings, including progress on my book. And I am grateful for my patient and loving husband, Eric, who does not care for medical dramas, yet has endured years of me talking about them. He and our beautiful children, Nora and Hazel, help me not to take life too seriously.

Preface

The Suspension of Disbelief and Medical Dramas

On May 9, 2002, I openly wept as I watched the final days of a trusted physician pass by. No, this was not a family member, or friend, or even a real person, but the fictional episode "On the Beach" of the television program *ER*, which chronicled the final days of the character Dr. Mark Greene. [1] And I was not alone. Approximately fifteen million people were tuning in at this time. [2] On fan sites, numerous viewers also admitted to being emotionally touched by the episode. For example, on TV.com, viewers called the episode "a tearjerker," and, many shared the sentiment of one poster who exclaimed, "This episode was so sad I was in floods of tears and I don't usually cry at anything!" [3] Like other popular television programs, *ER* made a lasting impression. Seven years later, at the end of its fifteenth season, an estimated 16.2 million people tuned in to bid farewell to the series. [4] Its popularity was reminiscent of another fictional medical program—*M*A*S*H*, the finale of which ranked as the highest viewed show of all-time, second only to the Super Bowl. [5]

Why are we so invested in these shows? What is it about medical dramas that have made them a constant of television? While other genres, like game shows, reality TV, and domestic sitcoms, have ebbed and flowed throughout history, medical dramas have been a part of television since *The Medic* in 1954. [6] We may switch out our McDreamy and (thankfully) have widened our definition of the TV health professional, but the reasons why we watch are not that different than sixty years ago—to witness these fictional docs heroically risk their careers and their lives to save us, the patients, as they battle microbes, bureaucrats, and other obstacles that emerge along the way.

And while most people will never experience the extreme situations presented in these shows, we can all relate and identify with the roles of the health care provider or the patient. While medical dramas are comprised of fictional storylines, their realism and authenticity has always been part of the appeal. Since the 1950s, producers have relied on real-life medical experts to ensure a degree of credibility.[7] Much more than other genres, fans have trusted the information in these programs.[8] And, while medical dramas are far from documentary looks at American health care, research has demonstrated that these shows can influence viewers' knowledge of medicine, perceptions of doctors and patients, and can even prompt audiences to adopt healthier lifestyle changes.[9]

Since television programs of this genre have appeared in each decade, they allow for a longitudinal exploration of television's distorted mirror, showcasing how Hollywood believed medicine should be presented to the general public, a perception that shifted over time. In this book, I explore how medical dramas have reflected, perpetuated, and, at times, challenged dominant ideologies in American society, tracing individualistic beliefs in health care to themes in these fictional programs. Ultimately, this book is about the fictional health professionals of these shows—typically the "heroic doctor"—a selfless healer, who goes above and beyond the job to counsel and save patients, regardless of the cost. At the same time, I emphasize the role of fictional patients in these storylines, whose often foolish behavior reinforces the knowledge and authority of the health care providers.

While this book is a critical analysis of medical dramas, I am also very much a fan, having viewed these programs long before I watched Dr. Greene live out his days on the beach. My fascination with fictional medical shows stems back to the first grade, when I witnessed paramedic John Gage suffer a rattlesnake bite while trying to save his patient in the 1970s show *Emergency!*. In elementary school, I tuned in weekly on Tuesday nights to William Shatner hosting the reenactment drama *Rescue 911*. My favorite episodes of sitcoms and other genres were the medical storylines, as I'll never forget when Punky Brewster needed her appendix removed or Will Smith was hospitalized for a gunshot wound in *The Fresh Prince of Bel-Air*. So when *ER* began in 1994, my freshman year of high school, I was hooked, and watched the program regularly for the next sixteen years. The profound impact of *ER*, *Chicago Hope*, *House, M.D.*, and *Grey's Anatomy* on my perceptions of the world prompted me to study these shows and their relationship to the changing messages in society. In other words, like so many other viewers, I have cheered for the heroic docs and laughed at the foolish patients.

NOTES

1. Wells, "On the Beach."
2. "We Look Back At The Top TV Shows of 2002."
3. "ER."
4. "Updated Thursday Ratings."
5. "Super Bowl 2010 Ratings."
6. Turow, *Playing Doctor*.
7. Ibid.
8. Davin, "Healthy Viewing."
9. Brodie et al., "Communicating Health Information Through The Entertainment Media"; Blumenfeld, "Some Correlates of TV Medical Drama Viewing"; Gerbner et al., "Health and Medicine on Television"; Chory-Assad and Tamborini, "Television Exposure and the Public's Perceptions of Physicians"; Glik et al., "Health Education Goes Hollywood"; "Television as a Health Educator."

Chapter One

The Health Responsibility Paradox and Televised Medical Dramas

In 2010, Congress passed the Patient Protection and Affordable Care Act (ACA), designed to extend health insurance benefits to all Americans.[1] This legislation was long overdue. By 2009, the uninsured population had grown to approximately fifty-seven million or 16.7 percent of Americans.[2] In addition, many Americans also face other economic consequences of the flawed system, including "job lock" (forced to stay at a position for fear of losing benefits) and "medical bankruptcy."[3] United States health care costs had skyrocketed, with expenses at 2.5 times per capita than the average spent in other wealthy countries, yet the quality of care was not better, just more expensive.[4]

Despite the necessity of affordable health insurance, uproar ensued over the mandates that Americans either acquire health insurance or pay a penalty.[5] Media played a significant role in the health care reform debates. A 2009 Pew Research Journalism study of 5,500 mainstream news stories found that health care dominated public discourse time.[6] Indeed, participants in the Kaiser Health Tracking Poll turned to media for information on the ACA, more than their doctors, employers, or insurance companies.[7] News on the political debates for health care reform were far from neutral. The Pew study identified much stronger language and themes in the news stories for those opposing reform than its supporters.[8] Furthermore, news offered little explanation about the implementation of the ACA, conveying confusing and contradictory messages that were politically-charged.[9] Such coverage may explain why so many Americans opposed the ACA, also referred to as "Obamacare."[10] Two years after the ACA was passed, only 47 percent of participants said that they approved of it.[11] Media and the American public regarded the ACA as a new concept, emerging with President Obama's administration. Yet, the notion of universal health care dates back to 1915 and was revisited by Presidents Eisenhower, Nixon, Carter, and Clinton.[12] Therefore, the ACA did not originate with President Obama, nor was it solely supported by the Democratic party.[13]

Given the historical precedence of universal health care, its bi-partisan support, and the overall benefits to the American public, why do so many people oppose the ACA? Some of the current opposition can be attributed to public confusion about the health care system and the middle and upper socioeconomic class' lack of first-hand experience with health care costs.[14] However, as Paul Starr argued, this resistance is much more complicated, stemming from American distrust in government and other institutions and above all, the tradition of individualism and agency entrenched in American culture. Starr wrote, "Only in the United States is public responsibility for health-care costs equated with a loss of freedom."[15]

Individualism has deep historical roots in American culture, with individual rights and accomplishments having been celebrated from at least the beginning of the nation.[16] This focus on individualism means that, as Robert Bellah explained, "Americans tend to think about their lives, values, independence and self-reliance above all else" and fits within the liberal democracy of the United States and myths of the "American Dream"—the notion that with hard work, anyone can achieve prosperity and success.[17] Indeed, our society rewards individual actions, with financial incentives for "good" choices, thus promoting individual responsibility. This culture of individualism encourages Americans to take charge of every aspect of their lives, through discourse that implicates individuals in creating their own happiness. This culture of individualism especially idealizes self-improvement in one's physical being. From improving one's eyesight with daily visual exercises to attempting to boost the immune system with Airborne, people are advised to modify nearly every aspect of their lives to maximize good health. Consumers are expected to take precautions to reduce risks of disease and injury by eating healthy foods, exercising regularly, practicing safe sex, and abstaining from smoking and illicit drugs. When people become sick or injured from "preventable" conditions (i.e., contract a sexually-transmitted disease), we tend to hold them more responsible than those with less "preventable" illness.

The emphasis on individualism extends to health professionals, who we hold responsible for providing quality medical care. With health care providers, a lapse in responsibility often translates to medical mistakes. Although errors have always occurred in medicine, a tradition of paternalistic doctor-patient relationships and a profession-wide fear of litigation have meant that most medical errors have gone unreported.[18] Yet heavy publicity of medical errors in the 1990s brought the issue of medical errors, and who should be held responsible for them, to the public's attention and prompted health officials to examine patient safety procedures. In 1999, the Institute of Medicine of the National Academies (IOM), a non-profit organization, produced a report defining and documenting the frequency and causes of medical errors.[19] In *To Err is Human: Building a Safer Health System*, the authors estimated that, nationwide, between 44,000 and 98,000 people die each year from medical errors—more than the number of deaths from traffic accidents, breast cancer or AIDS.[20] They also concluded that media attention focused far too much on individual health professionals, often ignoring institutional flaws in the American health care system.[21] With the publicity given to these findings, this study marked a pivotal moment: in the year 2000, a survey by the Kaiser Foundation found that 50 percent of Americans questioned knew of the IOM reports and their findings.[22]

Since the IOM findings and subsequent reports, stories of medical errors have been a staple part of popular media. For example, in 2007, numerous news outlets covered actor Dennis Quaid's experience with a nearly fatal medical error, in which his newborn twins were administered a medication 1000x the recommended dosage.[23] Yet even with the IOM research and the numerous popular media stories on medical errors, many people significantly underestimate the frequency of medical errors. For example, Blendon and colleagues found that 88 percent of physicians surveyed and 80 percent of the public thought that the number of deaths from medical errors per year was less than 50,000—half the number of deaths estimated by the IOM report.[24] And, despite the IOM's statements attributing most medical errors to institutional flaws, the majority of those surveyed believed that incompetent individual health professionals committed most medical mistakes.[25] Participants also believed patients to be "very often" responsible or "somewhat responsible" for medical errors.[26]

In theory, cleansing the American health care system of incompetent health professionals and teaching consumers about healthy choices benefits everyone. However, this emphasis on individuals has hindered institutional changes that would impact many more people than revoking the licenses of a few inept doctors or telling children to swap donuts for wheat toast. According to the IOM reports, most errors stem from institutional problems—the tradition of long hours for physicians and medical hierarchies that discourage others from questioning procedures, among other issues, situated within a fragmented health care system that impedes communication.[27] On the consumer side, the personal responsibility model has not been effective in significantly improving the health of Americans. Important issues remain unresolved—such as, why, for example, despite more than thirty years of health messages aimed at teaching people about heart-disease risk, obesity remains prevalent in the United States? Conflicting cultural messages likely hinder health promotion campaigns. Meredith Minkler explained that campaigns against childhood obesity, for example, likely fail because television bombards children with advertisements for junk food and discourages an active lifestyle, two recognized factors in childhood obesity.[28] The trend toward individual responsibility for one's health also assumes that all consumers are educated and therefore understand what precautions to take to prevent disease or injury, ignoring the fact that many people do not have the access, knowledge, or means to control their circumstances.[29]

The implications of the emphasis on individual responsibility for errors and good health are significant. This approach stigmatizes individual health professionals who make mistakes because of institutional flaws and blames consumers for becoming ill from a "preventable" condition. Even more importantly, this focus has created inherent opposition to the ACA and other health care reform that could significantly improve the nation's health. We are so accustomed to blaming individual consumers and health professionals that it is difficult to perceive problems with American health as a public domain issue.

THE ROLE OF MEDIA IN HEALTH CARE

Why has responsibility fallen to individual consumers and health professionals? This tradition helps explain much of the resistance to the ACA, as many people would rather live with a faulty health care system than sacrifice the "right" to make bad health choices. American media have reinforced and perpetuated individualism as part of the discord over health care reform, with stories and advice on self-improvement, paired with misleading myths about health care changes. Our perceptions of health care are shaped by personal, as well as vicarious experiences, much of which occur through mediated representations of reality. Information gleaned from popular media can shape consumer health decisions about when to visit a health professional, how to behave during a visit, and what treatment options one should choose.[30] According to Roxanne Parrott, "Media messages can be viewed as a kind of omnipresent third party whose influence is felt during the interactions that occur between health care personnel and clients."[31] In other words, even when people do not directly seek medical attention because of media content, previous media exposure may shape the overall medical process, from diagnosis to treatment, as well as how people perceive the roles of doctors and patients. In addition to publicizing legislative efforts about health care reform, news stories have highlighted individuals' roles in medical errors and preventative health. Robert Wachtner and Kaveh Shojania stated that the way that media generally report cases of medical errors suggests that mistakes could be easily reduced if "bad-apple physicians and nurses were purged, and sleep-deprived residents and interns were allowed to get a little shut-eye."[32] In other words, media have generally focused on individual flaws and not problems with the overall health care system, reinforcing the overall emphasis on individual responsibility for health. Popular media also emphasize the importance of the responsible health consumer. *WebMD* and other websites encourage self-diagnosis, news outlets tell of the latest preventative measures, and with the trend of pharmaceutical companies marketing directly to consumers, even advertisements advise people to request certain prescription drugs from their doctors.

Media coverage of health issues can also work as an agenda-setting tool. For example, heavy media coverage on the dangers of giving aspirin to children led to a dramatic decline in the incidence of Reye's syndrome.[33] A 1980s Kellogg's advertising campaign promoting the use of fiber in cancer prevention significantly boosted bran cereal purchases.[34] Similarly, news stories on First Lady Nancy Reagan's mastectomy in the mid-1980s led to an increase in breast-cancer patients choosing mastectomies over breast-conserving surgery.[35] And, following basketball icon Magic Johnson's announcement of his HIV status, survey research indicated increased public awareness of HIV risks and public willingness to get tested for sexually transmitted diseases.[36] Media messages about health can convey more than facts about a particular illness or condition. For example, Juanne Clarke found that while news magazines of the 1960s and 1980s presented cancer, heart disease, and AIDS as somewhat preventable, coverage of AIDS stigmatized people with the illness as shameful and the "scourge of society."[37] And Wang argued that health promotion advertising that uses disability to showcase the consequences of poor choices stigmatizes people with disabilities, portraying disability as a "fate worse than death.[38] Such stigma carries real-life implications, encouraging discrimination against people with stigmatized conditions and hindering Disability Rights activism.[39]

Cultural values and beliefs are entrenched in the media coverage of health issues. Jimmie Reeves and Richard Campbell suggested that 1980s media discourse about cocaine usage perpetuated many of the major political ideas of the Reagan administration.[40] Similarly, Jonathan Metzl explained how advertisements for psychotropic medications do not just convey drug information, but are "imbued with expectation, desire, gender, race, sexuality, power, time, reputation, countertransference, metaphor, and a host of important factors that a putative paradigm shift from interaction to prescription tacitly eliminates from psychiatry's purview."[41] These studies demonstrate that media coverage of health issues is not independent of political agenda or cultural biases, but draws from them to create the media story.

As network news audiences have declined, entertainment media have increasingly become an important tool in disseminating health information.[42] Joseph Turow asserted that fictional television can, in some cases, be more powerful than nonfiction media in helping people to understand institutions like medicine: "By acting out tales of life and death, of competency and immorality, in persuasive ways, TV fiction about health care can present compelling scenarios about what caregivers might do and what they should do when different types of people get sick."[43] Fictional television both reflects, perpetuates, and challenges dominant ideologies, which of course, shift over time. It is this cultural site that is the center of this book. Through the lens of entertainment television, I explore the interplay between media and culture in health care reform, tracing individualistic ideology through American history, with its distorted mirror in popular culture. This book focuses on the genre of medical dramas, which routinely model the doctor-patient relationships, and have been extensively proven to influence public perceptions of American medicine.[44] By examining the history of United States medicine, paralleled with media messages that have taught us about health care, shaped our perceptions of health professionals, and influenced our trust in the system, we can better understand the emphasis on individual responsibility over institutional change, and the resistance to legislation that provides solutions to an obviously flawed system.

Fictional portrayals of health care issues may be more digestible and appealing than debates about health care in nonfiction media content. George Annas argued that programs like *ER* and *Chicago Hope* "captured the public's imagination in a way that the Clinton Health plan never did" because of the fast-pace and visual appeal of the programs, as well as storylines that were easy to understand.[45] Particularly with medical dramas, which feature health professions, people learn about medicine—from terminology to salient health issues—from watching shows like *Marcus Welby, M.D., St. Elsewhere, ER,* and *Grey's Anatomy.* Medical dramas introduce viewers to such concepts as resuscitation orders, confidentiality, informed consent, do-not-resuscitate orders, and organ-donation release and let them "see" parts of the hospital that are typically off-limits to the public.[46] These programs portray the process of diagnosis, treatment, and outcome: viewers thus can learn not only from the narrative of the consequences of health decisions, but they also can see effects of choices as the dramas portray effects.[47] And viewers generally believe the messages in medical dramas, as demonstrated by Solange Davin, who found that some people were even less skeptical about the information presented in fictional television than in health documentaries.[48] Medical dramas can also encourage people to discuss health issues. One survey of *ER* viewers indicated that 51 percent talked with friends or family about health issues depicted on the show.[49] Furthermore, these programs can offer more than information, as depictions of illness can comfort sufferers of the disease by reminding them that they are not alone and may teach viewers what to expect during treatment for a specific disease.[50]

Educators have used medical dramas to teach students about diseases, treatment, and drug use, common health issues, appropriate physician behavior and patient interactions, as well as about the medical profession as a whole.[51] Truls Ostbye and colleagues used *ER* episodes in an epidemiology course to help students without health science backgrounds to learn about diseases, medical terminology, and coding forms, concluding that fictional television program can serve as an effective teaching tool.[52] Medical students have also used these programs to learn about health issues and the medical profession, including drug names, medical terminology, and appropriate physician behavior.[53] While at Harvard medical school, Dr. Ellen Lerner Rothman said that she and her classmates identified with the fictional medical students and residents in *ER*, and used the program to reinforce knowledge of clinical procedures and vocabulary:

> Through the *ER* physicians, residents, and medical students, my classmates and I explored who we wanted to be and what we were afraid we might become. We developed a paradigm for how we wanted to respond to our patients and explored how we would feel if we were unable to uphold it.[54]

Medical dramas have also influenced the popularity of specialties in medicine. Indeed, from 1994 (when *ER* began) to 1997, the rate of medical students applying to emergency medicine rose from 4 percent in 1994 to 5.2 percent in 1997.[55]

These programs are considered so influential that they are frequently used by public health advocates and scholars to promote issues as part of formal campaigns to disseminate health information and measure its effectiveness.[56] Researchers at the Kaiser Family Foundation helped *ER* writers create a storyline on emergency contraception.[57] After the episode aired, viewers were surveyed on their knowledge about the subject. Results indicated that 20 percent of the people surveyed first learned about emergency contraception from this particular episode of *ER*.[58] Overall awareness of emergency conception increased 17 percentage points for viewers, compared to knowledge of emergency contraception prior to the episode.[59] These scholars also surveyed viewers about their awareness of the Human Papilloma Virus (HPV)—a health issue discussed in an *ER* episode that first aired February 24, 2000.[60] Thirty-two percent of viewers first learned about HPV from the *ER* storyline, with the number of people who could provide accurate information about HPV tripling in the week after the episode aired.[61] Such "edutainment" has also been effectively used for other health purposes. Prosocial television messages helped successfully introduce the concept of the "designated driver," countered stigma about HIV and pregnancy through *Grey's Anatomy*, boosted awareness about immunizations, and influenced audience knowledge and behavior on a number of other health concerns.[62]

Medical dramas also impact public perception of physicians, the doctor-patient relationship, and the medical profession. Cultivation theory suggests that heavy viewers of television tend to see the world as it is presented in media.[63] Research has suggested that public confidence in the institution of medicine has changed with shifting portrayals of television physicians.[64] From the 1950s through the 1970s, when television depicted most doctors as heroes who rarely erred, in shows like *The Medic*, *Dr. Kildare*, and *Marcus Welby, M.D.*, heavy viewers trusted health professionals more than did light viewers or people who did not watch these programs.[65] As media portrayals of health professionals shifted over time, viewers' perceptions also changed. In the 1990s and 2000s, heavy viewers of television, especially "doctor shows," perceived physicians as less competent and credible than did light viewers.[66] At the same time, heavier viewers of prime-time medical programs believed physicians to be younger, more attractive, and more likely to be female than real-life socio-demographic data indicated.[67]

Research on medical dramas has been extensive, although narrow in scope: focusing on television portrayals of physicians and the public's perception of them. The textual studies have primarily used a systematic content analysis of television programs to determine general characteristics about physician depictions.[68] Qualitative analyses have also been more broadly focused—notably, Joseph Turow, Jason Jacobs, and Gregg Vandekieft, who provided histories of medical dramas, identifying shifts in the portrayals.[69] It is unclear, though, how and why these representations changed. This book aims to examine this gap in literature, exploring how the trend of individual responsibility has been reflected and perpetuated in popular discourse.

THE INTERPLAY BETWEEN CULTURAL PRODUCTS AND SOCIETY

This book is guided by the social construction of reality theory—the notion that our meaningful reality is shaped by media and other institutions.[70] Through constructed realities, like those in television, we learn our social roles, including those of health care provider and patient. Because social conventions and the language used to represent reality are so engrained in everyday life, most people are unaware of the existence of social constructions. As Peter Berger and Thomas Luckmann explained, "The man on the street does not ordinarily trouble himself about what is 'real' to him and about what he 'knows' unless he is stopped short by some sort of problem. He takes his 'reality' and his 'knowledge' for granted."[71] Literary theorist Raymond Williams wrote about the subtlety of social reality, which he calls "culture," stating, "A culture, while it is being lived, is always in part unknown, in part unrealized. The making of a community is always an exploration, for consciousness cannot precede creation, and there is no formula for unknown experience."[72] Sociologist Diana Crane also wrote about this "invisibility" of social reality, explaining that "in a sense, because it is 'embedded' in social structure, the influence of culture is often 'invisible' in realms of social life that are not depicted by the modern worldview as part of culture."[73] In other words, the ideologies that dominate media messages, like medical dramas, are so engrained in us, that we often take them for granted.

Crane suggested that embedded social realities are manifested in recorded culture (i.e., media products), and therefore, need to be studied, because, as she explained, "without analyzing the content and effects of recorded cultures as well as the factors that affect the content of recorded cultures, we cannot understand the role of culture in modern society"[74] Similarly, communications scholar James Carey equated studying recorded culture with understanding culture: "What can be called the study of culture can also be called the study of communications, for what we are studying in this context are the ways in which experience is worked into understanding and then disseminated and celebrated."[75] Thus, the study of medical dramas, as a site of recorded culture, provides a glimpse into the ideologies that have fueled American individualism and personal responsibility.

As part of constructing social realities, media convey and reinforce ideologies. Ideology has been defined in a number of ways, from the Marxist "false consciousness" to the more neutral conception of a "set of ideas."[76] Todd Gitlin articulated the media's role in reproducing ideologies:

> Commercial culture does not *manufacture* ideology; it *relays* and *reproduces* and *processes* and *packages* and *focuses* ideology that is constantly arising both from social elites and from active social groups and movements throughout the society (as well as within media organizations and practices).[77]

This research assumes that medical dramas reflect ideologies present in society, while they also focus and may reify them through storylines. And, when media and other institutions repeatedly reproduce particular ideologies, they can become part of a society's hegemony, referring to the dominance of one social group over others, which can produce a shared social understanding (common sense), as first defined by Antonio Gramsci.[78] Cultural Studies scholar Stuart Hall explained that "particular social groups struggle in many different ways, including ideologically, to win the consent of other groups and achieve a kind of ascendance in both thought and practice over them."[79] This consent is won through legitimation of particular ideas and the marginalization of countering ideas, and "the consent" becomes so engrained in culture that it appears "natural" or as "common sense." For this "common sense" to continue in society, ideas supporting the dominant power must be constantly disseminated and accepted in society. Hall asserted, "In order for one meaning to be regularly produced," it must "win a kind of credibility, legitimacy, or taken-for-grantedness for itself," and this involves "marginalizing, down-grading or de-legitimating alternative constructions."[80] Domi-

nant institutions like media, government, and religious and educational systems do not simply mirror society; they typically support and perpetuate a
culture's hegemony.[81]

As cultural sites, televised medical dramas can influence hegemonic systems by perpetuating or challenging prevailing ideologies. For example, in
the 1980s, J. Fred MacDonald argued that racial prejudices in American
culture had prevented African American actors from receiving central roles
in television programs.[82] Because television is a discursive site in which
dominant ideologies are reinforced or challenged, for an African American
actor to get to play a central role, such as a physician in a medical drama,
MacDonald declared, would require a "cultural transformation demanding
the abandonment of popular prejudices and the rejection of stereotypes."[83]
Since the time of MacDonald's statement, the type of people cast in medical
dramas have become much more diverse, expanding beyond Caucasian, able-
bodied, heterosexual, male physicians to include female and physicians of
color, as well as the representation of other groups. The casts of *ER* and
Grey's Anatomy have included Asian American, African American, British,
and Indian physician characters and characters with disabilities, with Drs.
Kerry Weaver in *ER*, Gregory House of *House, M.D.*, and Arizona Robbins,
who became an amputee after a plane crash in season nine of *Grey's Anatomy*. These examples demonstrate how representations in television may play
a role in reinforcing or challenging societal ideologies.

The medical dramas studied for this book repeatedly depicted fictional
interactions of health professionals and patients, and, as part of addressing
health issues in storylines, conveyed messages about responsibility. Because
messages addressed in televised medical dramas are linked to prevailing
ideologies about race, class, gender, and other social intersections, studying
these programs gives insight into ways in which the dominance of particular
social groups is reinforced, or challenged, in entertainment media. Attribu-
tions of health responsibility for fictional patients can support disparities of
power among social groups, reinforce or challenge stereotypes, and stigma-
tize members of a social group who are suffering from the depicted medical
condition. For example, popular media often stereotype African American
men as criminals. This stereotype has meant that, as a whole, this group is
perceived as less trustworthy and that, when a crime occurs, African
American men are usually blamed. Medical dramas may reinforce this
stereotype with storylines linking African American patients to criminal activity. For example, a fictional African American man needs surgery because
he was shot while robbing a convenience store. Medical dramas can challenge this stereotype with expanded roles for African American men (i.e., an
African American male professional with appendicitis) or with diversity in
the types of patients who require treatment due to gang violence (i.e., an
Asian female gang member).

Blaming individual fictional health professionals for mistakes can also convey messages about social dominance by suggesting what type of person is qualified to treat patients. At a time when all fictional physicians were Caucasian men, the types of physicians portrayed as fallible was not an issue because early medical dramas rarely included medical errors in storylines. As more diverse fictional physicians appeared, some of whom traditionally held dominant social positions, problems could appear in the type of fallible professional portrayed. For example, storylines that repeatedly feature only female health professionals making medical errors paint women as less qualified to treat patients than men. Since physicians have traditionally been male, showing flawed female professionals suggests that female doctors may be less skilled than male doctors and reinforces unequal power between men and women. This supports an ideology and societal structure of patriarchal hegemony.

Overall, this study assumes that all of a society's institutions, including media, play roles in shaping people's perceptions of responsibility. In turn, media products, such as medical dramas, draw from prevailing ideologies in society. The research reported in this book thus assumes that studying constructions of responsibility for health in medical dramas may give some insight into how and why individual responsibility for health has been emphasized in American society.

CONCLUSION

In recent decades, American society has placed responsibility for health primarily on individual consumers and health professionals. This emphasis on individual responsibility has meant that, for the most part, problems with the health care system have been overlooked, breeding medical errors and stigmatizing those who lack the resources needed to successfully reduce risks of disease or injury. This book examines how these constructions fit within the larger social trend of emphasizing individual responsibility for health through the following chapters.

To explore the contemporary trend of individual responsibility, this book addresses the history of American medicine and its depictions in art, including shifts in theories of disease causality, the rise of the health care system and the corresponding decline of public confidence in medicine. The foundation of this book was a textual analysis of 536 episodes of the programs *Chicago Hope*, *ER*, *House, M.D.*, and *Grey's Anatomy*. In addition to this research, 104 episodes of the earlier fictional medical programs *Marcus Welby, M.D.*, *M*A*S*H*, *Emergency!*, and *St. Elsewhere* were studied to provide context for the contemporary study.

In textual analysis, the meanings in these texts of medical dramas are not viewed as fixed but as shaped by ideas and values in American culture.[84] Peter Larsen explained that texts "express the general ideological trends (*Zeitgeist*) of a given period." Hence, knowledge of a culture helps to minimize "subjective' misinterpretations," according to Larsen, who argued that the text "should not be regarded as a closed segmented object with determinate, composite meanings, but rather as an indeterminate field of meaning in which intentions and possible effects intersect."[85] Klaus Bruhn Jensen stressed that media texts are historically situated, stating, "The language of textual sources, then, from legislation and business memoranda to newspapers, offers cues to how, for example, political and cultural rights have been conceived in different social and historical settings."[86] Therefore, as cultural products, media texts like medical dramas are shaped by prevailing ideologies in society and may give insight into prevailing ideologies and cultural trends about notions of responsibility, especially about health, in a society at the time.

Chapter two offers a brief history of the professionalization of medicine in America, from colonial times until the 1960s, correlating with the shifting representations of medicine. In chapter three, the rise of the personal responsibility model and its reflections in entertainment media is explored. This chapter focuses on the "heroic doctor" theme, a new configuration of the traditional depiction of physicians, in which the "docs" (or other health professionals) risk their careers or even lives to save their patients. These characters almost always cure their patients, regardless of their own numerous personal obstacles. Chapters four through seven use original research to explore contemporary representations of health professionals and patients in the medical dramas *Chicago Hope*, *ER*, *House, M.D.*, and *Grey's Anatomy*, examining, in chapter four, the flipside of the "heroic doctor" through an analysis of medical errors in these dramas. Chapter five explores fictional patients with "preventable" conditions, discussing how responsibility has been attributed to these characters. In chapter six, cases in which fictional patients were blamed for "non-preventable" conditions are discussed, looking at the negative depictions of "active" patients. Finally, chapter seven goes beyond the genre of medical dramas, examining constructions of health responsibility in other television programs and media sources, situating the popular discourse in this book within the contemporary landscape.

NOTES

1. Starr, *Remedy and Reaction*.
2. DeNavas-Walt, Proctor, and Smith, *Income, Poverty, and Health Insurance Coverage in the United States: 2010*.
3. Starr, *Remedy and Reaction*, 5.
4. Ibid.

5. Starr, *Remedy and Reaction.*
6. Staff, "What Americans Learned From the Media About the Health Care Debate."
7. 30 and 2013, "Kaiser Health Tracking Poll."
8. Staff, "What Americans Learned From the Media About the Health Care Debate."
9. Ibid.
10. Starr, *Remedy and Reaction*, 291.
11. Street et al., "Public Remains Split on Health Care Bill, Opposed to Mandate."
12. Starr, *Remedy and Reaction.*
13. Ibid.
14. Ibid.
15. Ibid., 9–10.
16. Bellah, *Habits of the Heart.*
17. Ibid., viii.; Wuthnow, *American Mythos.*
18. Gibson and Singh, *Wall of Silence the Untold Story of the Medical Mistakes That Kill and Injure Millions of Americans.*
19. America et al., *To Err Is Human.*
20. Ibid.
21. Ibid.
22. 01 and 2000, "Issues in the 2000 Election."
23. Jaffe, Barrett, and Shine, "Dennis Quaid Talks Medical Errors with Congress."
24. Blendon et al., "Views of Practicing Physicians and the Public on Medical Errors."
25. Ibid.
26. Ibid., 1937.
27. Campbell, Jr. and Cornett, "How Stress and Burnout Produce Medical Mistakes."
28. Minkler, "Personal Responsibility for Health?".
29. Ibid.
30. Parrott, "Advocate or Adversary?".
31. Ibid., 275.
32. Wachter and Shojania, *Internal Bleeding*, 20.
33. Soumerai, Ross-Degnan, and Kahn,, "The Effects of Professional and Media Warnings about the Association between Asprin Use in Children and Reye's Syndrome."
34. Levy and Stokes, "Effects of a Health Promotion Advertising Campaign on Sales of Ready-to-Eat Cereals."
35. Butler Nattinger, A. et al., "Effect of Nancy Reagan's Mastectomy on Choice of Surgery for Breast Cancer by US Women."
36. Basil, "Identification as a Mediator of Celebrity Effects."
37. Clarke, "Cancer, Heart Disease, and AIDS."
38. Wang, "Culture, Meaning and Disability."
39. Haller, *Representing Disability in an Ableist World.*
40. Reeves, Campbell, and Cambell, *Cracked Coverage.*
41. Metzl, *Prozac on the Couch.*
42. Wang, "Culture, Meaning, and Disability"; Soumerai, Ross-Degnan, and Kahn, "Effects of Professional and Media Warnings"; Street et al., "Key News Audiences Now Blend Online and Traditional Sources"; Singhal, *Entertainment-Education and Social Change.*
43. Turow, "Television Entertainment and the US Health-Care Debate."
44. Blumenfeld, "Some Correlates of TV Medical Drama Viewing"; Gerbner et al., "Health and Medicine on Television"; Chory-Assad and Tamborini, "Television Exposure and the Public's Perceptions of Physicians"; Brodie et al., "Communicating Health Information Through The Entertainment Media"; Glik et al., "Health Education Goes Hollywood"; "Television as a Health Educator."
45. Annas, "Reframing the Debate on Health Care Reform by Replacing Our Metaphors."
46. Turow, *Playing Doctor*; Gauthier, "Television Drama and Popular Film as Medical Narrative"; Davin, "Healthy Viewing: The Reception of Medical Narratives."
47. Gauthier, "Television Drama and Popular Film as Medical Narrative."
48. Davin, "Healthy Viewing: The Reception of Medical Narratives."
49. Brodie et al., "Communicating Health Information Through The Entertainment Media."

50. Sharf and Freimuth, "The Construction of Illness on Entertainment Television."

51. Turow, "Television Entertainment and the US Health-Care Debate."

52. Østbye, Miller, and Keller, "Throw That Epidemiologist out of the Emergency Room! Using the Television Series ER as a Vehicle for Teaching Methodologists about Medical Issues."

53. O'Connor, "The Role of the Television Drama ER in Medical Student Life."

54. Rothman and Rothman, White Coat: Becoming a Doctor at Harvard Medical School. 1st edition. New York: William Morrow Paperbacks, 2000.

55. Ibid.

56. Brodie et al., "Communicating Health Information Through The Entertainment Media."

57. Ibid.

58. Ibid.

59. Ibid.

60. Ibid.

61. Ibid.

62. Winsten, "Promoting Designated Drivers"; "Television as a Health Educator"; Glik et al., "Health Education Goes Hollywood."

63. Gerbner and Gross, "Living With Television."

64. Blumenfeld, "Some Correlates of TV Medical Drama Viewing"; Gerbner et al., "Health and Medicine on Television"; Chory-Assad and Tamborini, "Television Exposure and the Public's Perceptions of Physicians."

65. Blumenfeld, "Some Correlates of TV Medical Drama Viewing"; Gerbner et al., "Health and Medicine on Television."

66. Pfau, Mullen, and Garrow, "The Influence of Television Viewing on Public Perceptions of Physicians"; Chory-Assad and Tamborini, "Television Exposure and the Public's Perceptions of Physicians."

67. Pfau, Mullen, and Garrow, "The Influence of Television Viewing on Public Perceptions of Physicians."

68. McLaughlin, "The Doctor Shows"; Gerbner et al., "Health and Medicine on Television"; Pfau, Mullen, and Garrow, "The Influence of Television Viewing on Public Perceptions of Physicians"; Makoul and Peer, "Dissecting the Doctor Shows: A Content Analysis of ER and Chicago Hope"; Chory-Assad and Tamborini, "Television Doctors."

69. Turow, *Playing Doctor*; Jacobs, *Body Trauma TV*; Vandekieft, Gregg, "From City Hospital to ER: The Evolution of the Television Physician."

70. Berger and Luckmann, *The Social Construction of Reality*.

71. Ibid.

72. Williams, *Culture and Society 1780-1950*.

73. Crane, *The Sociology of Culture*.

74. Ibid., 3.

75. Carey, *Communication as Culture*, 44.

76. Eagleton, *Ideology*.

77. Gitlin, "Prime Time Ideology."

78. Hall, Evans, and Nixon, *Representation*.

79. Ibid.

80. Hall, "The Rediscovery of 'Ideology': Return of the Repressed in Media Studies."

81. Ibid.

82. MacDonald, "Black Doctors on Television."

83. Ibid., 151.

84. Larsen, "Textual Analysis of Fictional Media Content."

85. Ibid.

86. Jensen and Jankowski, *A Handbook of Qualitative Methodologies for Mass Communication Research*, 33.

Chapter Two

The Doctor: From Reaper to Hero

Early American Medicine and Its Shifting Representations

Contemporary attitudes toward health responsibility and choice did not simply appear with twenty-first century health care reform. While the knowledge and resources to prevent, diagnosis, and successfully treat disease have revolutionized medicine, today's attitudes can be traced back to the 1800s' theories of disease causality and a celebration of rugged individualism. This chapter explores the history of American medicine, examining its representations in art and literature—and later film and television. Such analysis of the past provides insight to the current social, political, and economic contexts as reflected and perpetuated in fictional and news media coverage.

EARLY HISTORY: MEDICINE AS A POOR-MAN'S TRADE

From colonial times until the late 1800s, many people did not consider physicians as especially trained or capable of curing disease. This social perception of doctors can be attributed to mistaken beliefs about disease etiology, the scarcity and poor quality of medical care in early America, and the popularity of lay healers—self-trained individuals who treated their families and neighbors.

The colonists had little access to trained physicians. Most skilled physicians were still practicing in Europe so the American colonists who provided medical care often derived their knowledge from reading books on medicine.[1] Any professional training was gained through an apprenticeship, usually in Europe.[2] Self-doctoring was common, as people cared for themselves and family members based on information they gleaned from medical guides. Clergymen also cared for the sick, as religion was deeply intertwined with medicine.[3] Since even those trained in medicine knew very little about what caused or could cure disease, most people attributed illness to a higher power.[4] Proponents of this supernatural theory believed that disease was God's punishment.[5] Since epidemics typically caused more deaths among the poor, people of the upper-classes used this theory to explain why disease occurred, arguing that those who were ill must have been "sinful" or "unworthy."[6] Besides supporting religious ideology, this theory of disease causality was also likely popular because it was believed to put no demands on the state service.[7]

To practice medicine in the United States in the 1800s, one did not need to hold a degree or license, although medical schools had been created by this time to train physicians. These schools were hardly rigorous. Because medical schools operated as commercial businesses, their operators focused on profit more than producing well-trained physicians.[8] To keep high enrollments, most medical schools had no admissions standards and admitted most Caucasian men who could afford schooling. In addition to schools for white men, nineteenth-century entrepreneurs created separate medical schools for African Americans and women.[9] On paper, medical schools claimed students would gain a basic knowledge of Latin and philosophy, serve a three-year apprenticeship, and write a thesis. However, most medical school operators did not strictly enforce these requirements.[10] Because medical licensing was not required, little could be done to prevent an incompetent physician from practicing.

Most physicians made little money from practicing medicine. Prior to the widespread construction of hospitals, doctors treated patients in their homes, or, less often, in the doctors' offices.[11] Due to transportation problems, physicians, especially in rural areas, could attend to very few patients in a single day.[12] Most people could not afford to spend much on medical care, so self-doctoring continued, as in colonial times, with the use of layperson's medical guides.[13]

Cultural attitudes also limited physicians' opportunities for profitable medical careers. Most people did not view physicians as authority figures.[14] The lack of cohesiveness among physicians, combined with the abundance of incompetent physicians, discouraged people from relying on doctors for "expert" opinions.[15] Democratic ideals also worked against making medicine an elite profession, especially during the 1830s Jacksonian era, which promoted egalitarianism.[16] As part of this emphasis on individual agency, people were encouraged to "take charge" of their health, as the "personal behavior theory" of disease causality became popular—a belief that one's actions influenced individual health.[17] To prevent or cure disease, some followers of this theory altered their diets to include more vegetables and botanical tonics.[18]

Others viewed hydropathy as therapeutic and vacationed at spas or mineral springs.[19] Clearly, this theory was designed for a privileged population. Sylvia Tesh explained how this approach to health was not feasible for members of the working class:

> To suggest to a textile worker in 1830 that her health depended entirely on changing her diet (when she barely had money to buy the cheapest foods), on access to copious amounts of water (when she hauled hers from a distant pump), or on her ability to relax in warm sunshine (when stress and overwork in crowded slums defined her life) was certainly obtuse and probably useless. Nevertheless, advocates of this theory of disease causality proclaimed its virtues to everyone.[20]

Two social movements in the 1830s popularized the personal behavior theory of disease causality, likely delaying more scientific approaches to medicine.[21] The Popular Health Movement, as called by scholars, grew out of an early women's movement and publicized the dangers of mainstream or "heroic" medicine, as some called it.[22] The leaders of this movement offered health education courses to women and advocated that women should use home remedies instead of risking a "trained" doctor's unsafe care.[23] At the same time, Samuel Thomas led the Thomasonian movement, aimed to democratize medicine by teaching people to become their own healers.[24] Its proponents argued that scientific medicine was often more detrimental to people's health than if they had no medicine at all.[25] By encouraging people to educate themselves about home remedies, this movement encouraged people to take responsibility for their health. And, as these two movements discouraged seeking a doctor's care, they undermined doctors who, at the time, already struggled to make a profit due to skepticism and a lack of trust in their medical skills. As with the supernatural theory of disease causality, the personal behavior theory placed the cause of disease on factors not connected to the environment, so the government was not expected to intervene with costly health reform.

Obviously, the personal behavior theory did not explain all disease or ill-health. In this 1800s era, other people attributed disease to environmental factors—a belief known as the miasma theory, which was popular intermittently from the Middle Ages until the 1800s.[26] Epidemics were often explained by this theory, particularly because they often occurred in crowded urban areas with poor sanitation.[27] Outbreaks of cholera, for example, were attributed to foul odors in the air.[28] Solutions then to the spread of disease included cleaning up city garbage, burying the dead in deep graves, and ventilating crowded rooms.[29] Thus, under the miasma theory, the government and other institutions were responsible for public health, by creating and maintaining a clean environment. For this reason, most politicians at the time did not favor the miasma theory, which was costly to the government.[30]

As with the personal behavior and supernatural theories, the miasma theory could be and was disproven.

LATE 1800S TO THE EARLY TWENTIETH CENTURY: THE GERM THEORY HELPS PROFESSIONALIZE MEDICINE

In the late 1800s, medicine began to radically change. Industrialization, medical innovation, and the popularity of rationalism, along with other economic, technological and social factors, helped to transform medicine from an unprofitable trade into an elite cohesive profession by the mid-twentieth century.

With industrialization, the population concentrations shifted from remote areas to cities. The boom of urban growth in the late nineteenth century brought new health concerns, and city officials struggled to control the overflowing garbage and sewage by providing waste removal and sanitary facilities.[31] Urbanization and transportation developments significantly decreased physicians' traveling time. Especially for rural physicians, the invention of the automobile made practicing medicine more profitable. With cars, doctors could visit many more patients in a single day, and patients with cars could get to their family physicians more quickly.[32]

Urban growth, combined with medical innovation, led to the construction of many hospitals. Until the early 1900s, charitable organizations typically funded hospitals to help the city's poor, who could not afford home-visits by doctors.[33] During this time, private hospitals had religious or ethnic affiliations. Jewish, Methodist, German, and similarly affiliated hospitals catered to members of their social groups and received extensive financial support from the community.[34] These hospitals provided medical, as well as spiritual, support to the "deserving poor"—those who had "fallen on hard times despite moral rectitude."[35] Non-deserving poor people ("drunkards," "sloths," or people who did not have social ties to a community) were treated at public or municipal hospitals, which had evolved from public almshouses.[36] Even at these "free" hospitals, patients paid nominal fees for their beds, under the belief of philanthropists that "paupers could easily slide into vice and criminality if allowed to abrogate responsibility to themselves and their dependents."[37] Due to the unsanitary conditions and lack of resources, both private and public hospitals had high mortality rates.

Nineteenth-century scientific discoveries contributed to changes in medicine by the early twentieth century. Aided by the creation of research institutions like Johns Hopkins University, in the 1800s, medicine advanced significantly. In the 1850s, anesthesia was first used in surgery, allowing patients to experience painless procedures, greatly expanding the amount of time surgeons had to operate.[38] As part of this era of innovation, scientists began questioning commonly-held perceptions about what caused disease, including the attribution of cholera to "foul air" (miasma). In 1854, a physician named John Snow traced the London cholera outbreak to contaminated water, demonstrating that foul air did not cause the outbreak.[39] Snow's discovery, along with the work of Louis Pasteur, Robert Koch and other scientists, set the stage for a new theory of disease causality.[40] In the late 1800s, scientists discovered that microorganisms existed and could cause illness.[41] Known as the "germ theory," this revelation explained why, even with praying to a higher power, bathing in natural springs, and spraying perfumes into the air (to get rid of odors), people were still getting sick. By understanding what caused disease, scientists, and later physicians, would learn how diseases could be transmitted.[42] With this knowledge, in 1867, Joseph Lister, a British surgeon, described the first antiseptic system for decreasing infection.[43] While it would take more than ten years for antiseptic practices to become standard in surgery, Lister's methods significantly decreased surgical mortality rates.[44] In the 1880s, the adoption of antiseptic practices greatly reduced high mortality rates from post-surgery infections.[45] Reducing the risk of infections also enabled surgeons to attempt new procedures, especially on the abdominal cavity, in which surgery had rarely been performed due to the extremely high rates of infection.[46] With clear evidence of the germ theory, other explanations of disease causality went out of favor, yet would resurface a century later, as medicine continued to change.[47]

With the new developments in medicine in the early twentieth century, it became standard practice for physicians to treat patients in hospitals. By 1910, physicians in hospital settings had access to diagnostic equipment and could perform complex antiseptic surgical procedures that could not be performed at home.[48] With the increase of wealthier patients needing hospital treatment, paired with the rise in urban migration, which often severed the migrants' community ties, most private hospitals opened their doors to clientele beyond those connected to the social affiliation of the hospital.[49]

The favorable publicity of the germ theory and other discoveries significantly improved public perception of physicians. By the 1900s, most people believed that (a doctor's) medical care was a necessary part of life.[50] With more people relying on trained physicians to treat their ailments, medicine became more profitable and shifted from a trade to a profession.[51]

By the turn of the twentieth century, when a number of trades, including law, had become established professions, more people turned to professionals for their specialized knowledge and skills. Higher standards for medical schools and medical licensing laws meant that fewer physicians graduated from medical school and became licensed to practice medicine.[52] These higher standards enhanced the status of those physicians who were able to graduate and attain licensure.[53]

As external factors made medicine more profitable, some people worked to make more rigorous standards for entry into the medical profession. Increased participation in the American Medical Association (AMA) and other associations helped to strengthen the profession of medicine as a network of physicians.[54] As medical practice became more specialized, doctors depended more on one another for referrals, which also unified physicians.[55] In the 1900s, people also aimed to standardize medical school training so that all medical students would graduate with the same set of skills and medical knowledge. In 1910, the Carnegie Foundation for the Advancement of Teaching hired Abraham Flexner to survey and rate 157 medical schools.[56] Flexner's report led to the closing of many weak schools, while remaining medical schools constructed lab facilities for research and raised admission standards.[57]

The professionalization of nursing also improved the quality of care in medicine. Traditionally, nursing was an occupation of the lower classes.[58] In the 1870s, women in the State Charities Aid Association organized a committee to oversee public hospitals and almshouses.[59] After observing poor sanitary conditions in these places, the women founded a training school for nurses, aimed at the middle class.[60] Since trained nurses could assist in complicated procedures and take on more challenging duties, professional nursing improved overall standards of care in medicine.[61]

One impediment to the standardization of medicine, however, was the dramatic drop in African American and female physicians. The Flexner report led to the closing of most of the medical schools for women and for African Americans because of poor ratings.[62] Mainstream medical schools became less open to admitting women and minorities, and the high cost of medical training discouraged even those who were accepted.[63] Licensing requirements reduced the role of lay healers, many of whom were women.[64] By the 1920s, medicine had become institutionalized, with organizational structures that "preserved a distinct sphere of professional dominance and authority."[65] For the most part, Caucasian men dominated this profession at this time.

In addition to improved medical treatments and facilities, new pharmaceutical control standards strengthened medicine as a profession. Before the early 1900s, people made significant profit by selling and distributing patent medicine, which was not only ineffective, but often contained harmful toxins.[66] In the early 1900s, muckraking journalists and Progressive Era reformers exposed deceptive business practices, especially the patent medicine industry, and advocated regulation.[67] At the same time, the increased finances and authority of the AMA enabled the association to launch its own attack against patent companies.[68] This fight for pharmaceutical regulation benefited from the patent companies' increased reliance on physicians for distribution.[69] In 1906, Congress passed the first Food and Drug Act, which required all statements on medicine bottles to be factual.[70] Although this law did not require pharmaceutical producers to disclose ingredients, nor regulate which drugs companies could distribute, it laid the foundation for the Food and Drug Administration, established in 1938, which tightened pharmaceutical regulation.[71]

By the 1930s, medicine had become a profitable, established profession and physicians were highly regarded by members of the public. Public-opinion polls from the Great Depression era indicated that people ranked medicine as the most prestigious profession, regardless of their own professions.[72]

EARLY TWENTIETH-CENTURY REPRESENTATIONS OF PHYSICIANS: FROM CARING TO CURING

Media messages have always reflected and perpetuated dominant perceptions of the health professions, which dramatically shifted as medicine changed from a trade to a profession. Until the late 1800s when medicine became a profession, physicians were not typically depicted as people who could cure disease.[73] Instead, artwork often depicted physicians as people who comforted those who were ill or dying.[74] An analysis of nineteenth-century physician depictions by Marc Cohen and Audrey Shafer suggested that artwork of the early 1800s illustrates the failure of doctors to cure their patients, explaining, for example, that Honoré Daumier's 1833 work *The Physician* depicted a doctor looking on helplessly as devils take his patients.[75] Such portrayals reinforced skepticism that physicians could heal their patients. News stories of the early 1800s also conveyed the mystery that surrounded disease. Journalism historian David Mindich noted that during the New York cholera outbreaks of 1832 and 1849, writers referred to both the miasma, personal behavior, and supernatural theories to explain the epidemics.[76] The abundance of disease causality theories, channeled through language loaded with biblical tales, demonstrated the lack of scientific knowledge about disease at this time.[77] Overall, popular culture products and news suggested and reinforced the ineptitude of physicians at a time when they could do little to heal patients.

As medical practice became a credible and elite profession, artistic portrayals of physicians changed. Beginning in the late 1800s, as medical innovations enabled physicians to treat significantly more ailments, artwork increasingly depicted the physician as the "keeper and developer of a new knowledge," according to Cohen and Shafer.[78] From the 1880s until the mid-twentieth century, most portrayals of medicine in artwork focused on medical procedures and technology more than on the treating physician, as highlighted in Raoul Dufy's 1930 drawing titled *The Operation,* which focused on the surgical procedure more than the physicians performing it.[79] Likewise, newspapers of the late 1800s also indicated a shift in perceptions of medicine and in science. Mindich described how newspaper coverage of the 1866 cholera outbreak differed greatly in tone and ideology than the earlier epidemics.[80] Instead of attributing the disease to God's wrath or personal inadequacies, writers mentioned the source of cholera ("the excreta"), framed through an objective lens that highlighted, as Mindich stated, "scientific investigation."[81]

Advertising also heavily promoted this faith in scientific authority. During the 1800s, the mass production and marketing of products made advertising a profitable enterprise, particularly for drugs, tonics, and other concoctions.[82] Since both advertising and pharmaceutical manufacturing were unregulated at this time, people could sell whatever potions they created, making outrageously false claims about its healing properties.[83] Marketed through traveling "medicine shows," magazines, newspapers, patent medicine catalogs and other sources, people purchased these "remedies" for nearly any ailment, from toothaches to consumption, which often contained morphine, cocaine, high percentages of alcohol, or laxatives.[84] In the early 1900s, the creation of the Food and Drug Act and another regulation greatly reduced patent medicine products. However, the reliance on medicine to treat or cure illness that developed during the patent medicine era became a staple part of American culture, helping to establish physicians as authority figures. The doctor's status would only become more elevated in the next era, aided by popular culture representations.

1940S–1960S: "THE GOLDEN AGE OF MEDICINE"

During the years from the 1940s to the 1960s, an era that scholar John Burnham labeled "the Golden Age of Medicine," the public generally had high regard for people in the medical profession.[85] By the 1940s, the medical innovations of the turn of the century, in addition to medical progress of the 1920s and 1930s, such as the discovery of penicillin, had significantly improved the quality of medicine. Between the 1940s and the 1960s, the development of effective antibiotics, vaccines for a number of deadly and crippling illnesses, including tuberculosis and polio, and significant surgical advancements, such as organ transplants, continued to improve patient care. In this era, people generally trusted physicians, believing that they usually acted in the patients' best interests.[86]

With the introduction of health insurance programs, by mid-century, access to medical treatment significantly improved. In the 1940s, most employers began offering group health insurance for their employees.[87] Since medical procedures were relatively inexpensive, insurance was fairly affordable for most of the population.[88] In turn, because most of the population had access to health insurance, politicians largely ignored the notion of developing programs for the uninsured. Therefore, people who could not afford insurance had few options, especially without the charity hospitals and inexpensive health care that had been available in previous years.[89]

In the 1950s and 1960s, some efforts were made to provide insurance to the uninsured. As part of the Civil Rights Movement, some reformers questioned the implication of the poor in their own impoverishment. As opposed to traditional beliefs that people became poor because they lacked a work ethic, liberal reformers cited cultural reasons for poverty, such as racism and violence.[90] In this view, poor people were blameless victims, "condemned to a life of poverty by forces quite beyond their own control," according to Jonathan Engel.[91] In response to changing cultural attitudes toward poverty and growing concern about the elderly, President Lyndon Johnson approved Medicare as part of the Social Security Act in 1965, which provided insurance for those aged 65 and older and for people with disabilities, and Medicaid, providing insurance for low-income families.[92]

During the 1940s through the 1960s, the germ theory continued to dominate as the primary theory of disease causality. This was an era of optimism for American medicine. While research first linked individual behavior to health in the 1950s (with smoking to cancer), it would be several decades before the germ theory's popularity would diminish. As the following section explains, the focus on individual behavior, however, did not become prevalent in political and public discussions until the 1970s.

DEPICTIONS OF THE DOCTOR AS A COMPASSIONATE HERO

In the first half of the twentieth century, depictions of medicine typically focused on the technology and procedures used to treat patients. However, some members of the public began to feel that the new system of medicine was impersonal and that physicians were emotionally detached from their patients. In response to this public concern, images that focused on medical technology declined as artwork began to feature physicians, showing them as caring and skilled healers.[93]

From the 1930s through the 1950s, film (and later) television often portrayed doctors in their storylines, conveying images of caring and compassionate doctors who skillfully used medical technology to perform complex procedures.[94] Since physicians traditionally were important figures in most societies, screenwriters could easily fit a physician character into different time periods and cultures.[95] Regardless of the genre or time period in which the film or program was set, doctors were typically depicted as caring and knowledgeable. For example, the *Doctor Kildare* films of the 1930s and

1940s exemplify the typical portrayal of a doctor at this time—an infallible compassionate hero dedicated to saving lives regardless of the cost.[96]

The physician character appeared early in television history. In 1954, the television program *The Medic* became the first successful medical drama.[97] As had been true in films earlier, heroic doctors in this television program seldom failed to cure their patients.[98] This trend continued throughout the 1950s and 1960s, most notably with programs like *Doctor Kildare* (featuring characters from the film series), *Ben Casey*, and *Marcus Welby, M.D.* The drama *Medical Center* (1969–1976) especially featured infallible doctors. Even more so than in other television medical dramas, physicians in this program cured nearly all of their patients.[99] According to Gregg Vandekieft, the success rate of fictional physicians in 1960s medical dramas reflected political attitudes, as most people believed that the "established institutions were engines of social good" that worked in the public's best interest.[100] Therefore, the heroism of fictional doctors during this era reflected the general optimism toward institutions as a whole.

The heroic doctor image dominated medical dramas from early television to the 1970s. In a content analysis of television at this time, James McLaughlin found that almost all television physician characters were young or middle-aged, Caucasian, and male and frequently used high risk or experimental procedures to save their patients.[101] He described the "typical" TV doctor as "powerful, almost omnipotent, healer who performs his duties above and beyond normally expected capacities. He does so in situations that are exciting or controversial and deals with not only the physical but also the emotional needs of his patients."[102] Similarly, as part of the Cultural Indicators research, Gerbner and colleagues analyzed 10 years of dramatic television content (over 1600 programs) and three years of commercials to examine how television portrayed health professionals, the health profession and physical injury, illness and risk factors, such as obesity, safety, smoking and drinking.[103] Gerbner and colleagues found that television depicted doctors as "a bit more fair, sociable, and warm than most characters" and that they were portrayed as "smarter, more rational, more stable, and fairer than nurses."[104] Medical dramas focused on doctors, not other types of health professionals.

Such positive portrayals were likely influenced by the involvement of the AMA. Members played a prominent role in determining the content, medical terminology, and patient outcome depicted in the dramas during the 1940s–1960s by routinely revising and approving the scripts, as each program had a medical professional who advised writers on medical issues and terminology.[105] Real-life physicians, however, had mixed feelings about their on-screen counterparts during this era of heroic fictional doctors. Some doctors praised television medical dramas for offering positive representations of medical professionals, while others criticized Kildare, Casey, and Welby for offering unrealistic depictions, arguing that they had unbelievable cure rates.[106] Physicians also disapproved of representations of doctor-patient relationships, suggesting that the amount of time physicians spent with each patient and the efforts doctors invested in their patients gave the public unrealistic expectations about patient care.[107] For example, physicians criticized the format of *Marcus Welby, M.D.*, claiming that Welby devoted too much time to a single patient, painting a false picture of the family physician.[108]

Despite this criticism, heroic doctor characters have always been popular with audiences. The character Dr. Kildare appeared in more than nine films and a long-running television series. *Medical Center* and *Marcus Welby, M.D.* each ran for seven seasons. These programs and their successors heavily influenced how people perceived physicians and the health profession as a whole. An early study of the influence of fictional medical dramas on public perception of the medical profession suggested that heavy viewing of shows like *Ben Casey* and *Dr. Kildare* resulted in a "positive attitude toward physicians."[109] Peter Sandman argued that viewers of "doctor shows" learned that doctors should be heroes who "sacrifice their personal lives and personal relationships to the welfare of their patients."[110] Thomas Volgy and John Schwarz reported that heavier viewers of television have more positive attitudes toward physicians than do light viewers.[111] And, of course, Gerbner and colleagues' landmark cultivation research also supported this relationship, noting that people who watch more television have higher confidence in doctors than those who watch less.[112] This correlation may have even been more pronounced by 1980, in that real-life attitudes toward health care had become noticeably negative.[113]

Overall, visual representations shifted along with the growing professionalization of medicine in the late 1800s to portray doctors as nearly God-like healers who would do anything for their patients. This image would dominate entertainment for most of the twentieth century. However, as the following chapter explains, in the late 1970s and 1980s, a more humanized physician would replace its infallible predecessor. Yet, even within this darker version, TV's docs would continue to save their patients.

NOTES

1. Cassedy, *Medicine in America.*
2. Starr, *The Social Transformation of American Medicine.*
3. Cassedy, *Medicine in America.*
4. Starr, *The Social Transformation of American Medicine.*
5. Tesh, *Hidden Arguments.*
6. Ibid.
7. Ibid.
8. Barry, *The Great Influenza.*
9. Starr, *The Social Transformation of American Medicine.*
10. Ibid.

11. Ibid.
12. Ibid.
13. Ibid.
14. Ibid.
15. Ibid.
16. Ibid.
17. Tesh, *Hidden Arguments*.
18. Ibid.
19. Ibid.
20. Ibid., 23.
21. Ehrenreich and English, *For Her Own Good*.
22. Ibid.
23. Ibid.
24. Ibid.
25. Ibid.
26. Tesh, *Hidden Arguments*.
27. Ibid.
28. Johnson, *The Ghost Map*.
29. Tesh, *Hidden Arguments*.
30. Ibid.
31. Cassedy, *Medicine in America*.
32. Starr, *The Social Transformation of American Medicine*.
33. Ibid.
34. Ibid.
35. Ibid., 9.
36. Ibid.
37. Ibid., 11.
38. Starr, *The Social Transformation of American Medicine*.
39. Johnson, *The Ghost Map*.
40. Gaynes, *Germ Theory*.
41. Ibid.
42. Ibid.
43. Ibid.
44. Ibid.
45. Starr, *The Social Transformation of American Medicine*.
46. Ibid.
47. Tesh, *Hidden Arguments*.
48. Engel, *Poor People's Medicine*.
49. Ibid.
50. Burnham, "American Medicine's Golden Age: What Happened to It?".
51. Starr, *The Social Transformation of American Medicine*.
52. Ibid.
53. Ibid.
54. Ibid.
55. Ibid.
56. Cassedy, *Medicine in America*.
57. Ibid.
58. Starr, *The Social Transformation of American Medicine*.
59. Ibid.
60. Ibid.
61. Ibid.
62. Ibid.
63. Ibid.
64. Ehrenreich and English, *For Her Own Good*.
65. Starr, *The Social Transformation of American Medicine*, 27.
66. Starr, *The Social Transformation of American Medicine*.

67. Ibid.
68. Ibid.
69. Ibid.
70. Hilts, *Protecting America's Health.*
71. Ibid.
72. Raben, "Men in White and Yellow Jack as Mirrors of the Medical Profession."
73. Cohen and Shafer, "Images and Healers: A Visual History of Scientific Medicine."
74. Ibid.
75. Ibid.
76. Mindich, *Just the Facts.*
77. Ibid.
78. Cohen and Shafer, "Images and Healers: A Visual History of Scientific Medicine," 201.
79. Cohen and Shafer, "Images and Healers: A Visual History of Scientific Medicine."
80. Mindich, *Just the Facts.*
81. Ibid.
82. Anderson, *Snake Oil, Hustlers and Hambones.*
83. Ibid.
84. Ibid.
85. Burnham, "American Medicine's Golden Age: What Happened to It?".
86. Ibid.
87. Laham, *A Lost Cause.*
88. Engel, *Poor People's Medicine.*
89. Ibid.
90. Ibid.
91. Ibid., 21.
92. Cohen and Shafer, "Images and Healers: A Visual History of Scientific Medicine."
93. Ibid.
94. Ibid.
95. Shale, Richard, "Images of the Medical Pofession in the Movies."
96. Turow, *Playing Doctor*; Vandekieft, Gregg, "From City Hospital to ER: The Evolution of the Television Physician."
97. Turow, *Playing Doctor.*
98. Ibid.
99. Vandekieft, Gregg, "From City Hospital to ER: The Evolution of the Television Physician."
100. Ibid., 220.
101. McLaughlin, "The Doctor Shows."
102. Ibid., 184.
103. Gerbner et al., "Health and Medicine on Television."
104. Ibid., 902.
105. Turow, *Playing Doctor.*
106. Ibid.
107. Ibid.
108. Ibid.
109. Blumenfeld, "Some Correlates of TV Medical Drama Viewing," 902.
110. Sandman, "Medicine and Mass Communication," 381.
111. Volgy and Schwarz, "TV Entertainment Programming and Sociopolitical Attitudes."
112. Gerbner et al., "Health and Medicine on Television."
113. Shore, *The Trust Crisis in Healthcare.*

Chapter Three

"I have my hand on a bomb. I'm freaking out. And most importantly, I really have to pee."

American Health Care, 1970–2000s, and Its Flawed Heroes

By the 1970s, the Golden Age of Medicine had come to an end.[1] Changes in cultural attitudes, skyrocketing health care costs, and reform that depersonalized the doctor-patient relationship dramatically shifted how people perceived health professionals and the medical profession.[2] How could the heroic doc survive in an era of public distrust and cynicism? This chapter outlines the contemporary history of American medicine, describing the rise of the personal responsibility model, and its changing representations.

1970S–1980S: PREVENTIVE MEDICINE, PERSONAL RESPONSIBILITY, AND THE RISE OF HMOS

In the course of the twentieth century, medical innovations had greatly expanded the role of medicine, from curing to preventing ill health. In 1900, the average life expectancy was 47.3 years.[3] Seventy years later, the average life expectancy had increased to 70.8 years.[4] With most of the population living longer, scientists and health professionals began to investigate ways to prevent, not just treat, medical conditions.[5]

In 1950, Sir Austin Bradford Hill, an English epidemiologist, discovered that people who smoked more cigarettes were disproportionately more likely to develop lung cancer.[6] This connection not only demonstrated the dangers of smoking, but also scientifically proved that individual behaviors could impact health.[7] Hill's research spurred research examining other links between behavior and health, which led to the development of the personal responsibility model—a theory of disease causality in which individual choices impact health.[8]

During the 1960s, politicians began to address preventive medicine and the role of individual behavior in health. A 1961 speech at the National Health Forum illustrates this transition, as New York City Department of Health Commissioner Leona Baumgartner declared, "We are passing from a medicine in which you do something to the patient into medicine in which we must do something with the patient and in which he must do a lot more on his own."[9] And, based on Hill's research about the dangers of cigarettes, in 1964, President Johnson warned consumers that smoking was dangerous to one's health, prompting the FDA to require all cigarette packages to contain warnings about the risks of smoking.[10]

By the 1970s, health policy experts and health professionals began to emphasize to consumers the importance of making healthy choices. Reminiscent of the personal behavior theory in the 1830s, this approach advised consumers to make good lifestyle choices to reduce their risk of disease. The popularity of the personal responsibility model made sense in a decade that celebrated individualism. As part of the Civil Rights and Feminist movements, people were encouraged to question authority, including medical authority, and to become more active in their health.[11] Legislation aided the shift in the doctor-patient model. Although the notion of "informed consent" had been in place since the 1950s, doctors often failed to advise patients of surgical risks.[12] In 1972, the U.S. Supreme Court ruled that all physicians were required to explain medical procedures and discuss all potential risks.[13] With medicine becoming less paternalistic between doctor and patient, people began to view medical treatment as a partnership in which patients were encouraged to ask questions about their medical conditions and share in decisions about treatments.[14] The personal responsibility model complemented the "active" patient model by encouraging people to take control of their health.

In 1979, the personal responsibility model was established as the primary guide for American health policy when the U.S. Department of Health, Education, and Welfare released a report emphasizing the importance of individual behavior.[15] Titled *Healthy People*, this report declared, "It is the controllability of many risks—and often, the significance of controlling even only a few—that lies at the heart of disease prevention and health promotion" and outlined ways in which individuals could reduce stress, improve diets, and develop exercise plans.[16] This report established objectives for reducing coronary disease, lung cancer, and strokes in America, as well as for reducing traffic fatalities and drug use among adolescents.[17] While the authors recognized that personal behavior did not guarantee good health, it emphasized the importance of good choices, stating, "Healthy behavior, including judicious use of preventive health care services, is a significant area of individual responsibility for both personal and family health."[18] This document marked the beginning of the dominance of the personal responsibility model, which would guide United States health policy for at least the next thirty years.

In addition to changing cultural attitudes toward medicine, medical innovation was changing the health care system of the 1970s. By this time, medical and surgical treatments for illness and injury had dramatically increased and health professionals were able to perform open heart surgery, transplant kidneys and other organs, and diagnose some congenital diseases before childbirth, among other new procedures.[19] While these innovations improved the overall health of America, they also dramatically increased the cost of medical treatment and subsequently, insurance premiums.[20] National health insurance was proposed to alleviate the cost—a plan supported by U.S. presidents Richard Nixon and Jimmy Carter, the Health Insurance Association of America (HIAA), and, to some extent, the AMA.[21] However, national insurance was not widely supported by the general population, likely because 87 percent of Americans had health insurance.[22] Because of the lack of public support, combined with fears that a national health insurance program would contribute to the existing problem of inflation and worsen the federal deficit, no national health insurance programs were seriously considered in the 1970s.[23] Instead, Congress approved the Health Maintenance Organization Act of 1973, allowing the use of cost-sharing among a network of providers.[24] Health Maintenance Organizations (HMOs) became gatekeepers, limiting access to certain health care providers and forcing people to switch primary physicians, undermining the doctor-patient relationship.[25] As the rise of HMOs made health insurance a profitable business, many people came to see these companies as corporate entities that sacrifice the quality of patient care for profit.[26] And, as part of reducing health care costs, the personal responsibility model became the dominant ideology for public health, a cost-effective measure, given that the promotion of individual-level changes was far cheaper than an overhaul of the health care system itself.[27] This distrust in HMOs, paired with the 1970s questioning of authority and emphasis on individual responsibility, began to erode public confidence in the overall health care system.[28]

In the 1980s, a political backlash to the social movements of the previous two decades ensued as the Reagan administration implemented political, social, and economic changes that attempted to undo equal rights victories of the previous two decades.[29] Conservatives also advocated a return to traditional family structures and values, with the election of President Ronald Reagan. As part of his platform, President Reagan prided himself on his dedication to preserving family values.[30] Yet many of the 1970s issues in health care continued in the 1980s, including the rise of HMOs to combat health care costs escalating, partially due to the development of expensive diagnostic equipment, including CT scans, ultrasound machines, and MRI scanners.[31] These increased costs prompted many employers to reduce or eliminate health insurance plans.[32]

In the 1980s, objectives of the 1979 *Healthy People* report were carried out in numerous health promotion campaigns. In addition to anti-smoking campaigns popularized in the previous decade, 1980s health campaigns promoted other healthy behaviors, such as choosing healthy food, exercising, and using seatbelts and helmets to prevent injury.[33] The Reagan administration also furthered the emphasis on personal responsibility by reducing the budget for many health programs, placing responsibility for health on individuals.[34] Writing in 1981, John Allegrante and Lawrence Green criticized the health policies of the Reagan administration, warning that the "government must not abandon its proper role in regulating or subsidizing social conditions that mitigate or support behavior conducive to health."[35]

The rise in HMOs, paired with budget reductions in health programs, caused trust in the health care system to further decline. According to Allegrante and Green, many people in the 1980s viewed medical care as "being costly, unresponsive, overly technologized, and bureaucratic."[36] Overall, in the 1980s, public skepticism about health professionals and the medical profession mounted due to increased enrollment in HMOs, budget cuts affecting health programs, and policies that reflected an emphasis on individual responsibility for health.

CONFLICTING PORTRAYALS: THE HEROIC "WISE GUY" DOCTOR AND THE FLAWED PROFESSIONAL

Television content of the 1970s and 1980s reflected the changes in attitudes toward health professionals and the medical profession. As opposed to earlier medical dramas, which portrayed physicians as infallible compassionate heroes, television in the 1970s and 1980s did not always portray physicians positively. Medical dramas of this era offered conflicting messages about medicine and health professionals.

In many ways, medical dramas of the 1970s and 1980s continued generic conventions of earlier eras. The army dramedy *M*A*S*H* and its spin-off *Trapper John*, the paramedic drama *Emergency!* and *St. Elsewhere* all primarily featured handsome, Caucasian men with Hawkeye Pierce, Trapper John, and Henry Blake in *M*A*S*H*, Drs. Brackett and Early in *Emergency!*, and seven of the original physician characters in *St. Elsewhere*. And, as with the traditional heroic TV doc, these physicians were professionally infallible—the health professionals cured most patients and had very low morbidity and mortality rates. Even *M*A*S*H*, which was set at an army hospital during the Korean War, appeared to have surprisingly high survival rates. We also saw a continued paternalism in the fictional doctor-patient relationship. The programs focused on the doctors, with patients playing minor roles in the storyline. In *Emergency!*, most conversations about the patients took place without the patient present. Most patients in *M*A*S*H* were unconscious, therefore, not part of the decision-making process. And in *St. Elsewhere*, even when doctors explained diagnosis, the prescribed treatment was not presented as a choice. For example, Dr. Craig tells an obese patient that he can decide whether or not to have surgery, but if he elects not to, he will die very soon. Programs of other genres, such as *The Cosby Show, Doogie Howser, M.D.,* and *Northern Exposure,* also offered positive depictions of physicians, featuring likeable, competent physicians. [37]

At the same time, medical programs of this era challenged the formula of the traditional medical drama, beginning with *M*A*S*H* (1972–1983). Unlike the earlier medical dramas set in American hospitals and clinics, *M*A*S*H* took place at an army hospital during the Korean War, often addressing social and political issues of the time. In many episodes, the doctors experienced the devastation of war, as exemplified with the death of Colonel Henry Blake, who is killed in a plane crash after he is discharged. This program was also the first to show doctors and nurses with personal and often humorous problems. Gregg Vandekieft explained the personal flaws of the lead character, Dr. Benjamin Franklin "Hawkeye" Pierce, describing him as "an iconoclast who drank heavily, womanized, and lacked the typical accoutrements of professional demeanor."[38] With characters like Hawkeye, *M*A*S*H* was the first to blend humor with drama in a medical program. Doctors in this program regularly played pranks on the other characters and consistently made jokes about them.[39] Yet, inside the operating room, the doctors and nurses consistently demonstrated their exceptional skills, despite the harsh conditions of the army hospital.

Like *M*A*S*H*, *St. Elsewhere* (1982–1988) depicted health professionals who were cynical and flawed people, many of whom had more problems than their patients.[40] Over its six-season run, some of the physicians depicted in *St. Elsewhere* were promiscuous, obese, and bumbling.[41] Storylines included a plot in which nurses shoot a physician who rapes women, a bulimic doctor commits suicide, and a pathologist engages in sexual intercourse in the hospital's morgue.[42] Even with all of these personal obstacles, for the most part, the health professionals continue to provide excellent care for their patients. In this time period, *The Cosby Show* was the first in television history to feature an African American physician as a central character, challenging the stereotype of the traditional physician as a Caucasian man. It should be noted, however, that practicing medicine was usually peripheral to other events in the program, much like portrayals of medical professionals in *The Donna Reed Show* in the 1950s and 1960s.[43]

Medical dramas of the 1970s and 1980s were also slightly more diverse than the homogenous Caucasian programs of the past. During this time, the medical profession became much more diverse as actions from the Civil Rights and Feminists movements prompted women and people of color to attend medical school. In 1970, only 9.2 percent of medical school graduates were female.[44] By 1985, the number of female medical school graduates had risen to nearly 31 percent.[45] The number of people of color in medical school also grew.[46] While people of color and women appeared in guest roles and as minor characters in *M*A*S*H* and *Emergency!*, *St. Elsewhere* had a much more diverse cast than previous medical dramas, including both female and African American physicians in positive portrayals. However, despite progress in the quantity and quality of roles for underrepresented groups in medical programming, scholars argued that these programs still offered limited roles for people of color.[47]

Overall, television negotiated the changing public attitudes toward health care with conflicting portrayals of the profession. The personally flawed, but still heroic, doctor likely offered audiences humanized characters, with whom they could identify, while preserving the omnipotent fictional healers of television. As with earlier shows, though, patients continued to play minor, almost nonexistent, roles in the storylines, which would change with the next era of medical dramas.

1990S–2000S: THE FAILURE OF "HILLARYCARE" AND THE RISE OF MANAGED CARE PLANS

By the 1990s, health care costs had become a salient issue in the political arena. Many businesses had eliminated health care plans for employees and by 1992, approximately nineteen million people were uninsured.[48] And changes in government funding during the 1980s also left Medicare recipients with less coverage than before.[49] In addition to the growing number of people without insurance, social changes increased the need for health care reform. For example, in the 1980s and 1990s, more children were born out of wedlock and raised by single parents than ever before in the United States, and these trends correlated with increased poverty and poorer health care.[50]

As noted, the notion of universal health care coverage was discussed during earlier political administrations.[51] Yet the Clinton administration's focus on health care reform, at a time in American history in which many were without health insurance, resulted in heavily publicized debates that had not occurred during other presidencies.[52] After his first election, Clinton quickly established the Task Force on National Health Care Reform, a committee designed to develop a universal health care plan, headed by First Lady Hillary Rodham Clinton.[53]

Presented before Congress in 1993, the "HillaryCare" plan, as it was nicknamed, mandated health care for employees through government regulated HMOs.[54] Republicans, members of the Health Insurance Association of American, and others heavily criticized the plan, claiming that it was too bureaucratic and restrictive for patients.[55] Some members of the AMA also opposed the plan, arguing that the Health Security Act would decrease physician fees and limit the services a doctor could perform.[56] The Republican Party gained control of Congress in the 1994 election, marking the end of serious consideration of universal health care.

At this time, managed care plans were implemented across America. Rising costs and the promises of what managed care plans could achieve encouraged many hospitals to enroll in either the preferred provider organization or HMOs.[57] As Jeffrey Bauer pointed out, this system had many flaws. Because this system was focused on streamlining the costs of health care, it did not allow more people to gain health insurance, nor did it improve the quality of patient care.[58] In fact, under managed care, many people, both insured and uninsured, were denied treatment for medical conditions that would have been approved in previous years.[59]

For the health care industry, however, the implementation of managed care was lucrative. The reduced coverage for patients and negotiated discounts with providers meant that managed care plans yielded exceptional profits.[60] Some scholars argued that Clinton's health care reform likely failed because of the financial support politicians received from the health care industry.[61] Since managed care plans were more profitable than universal health care, many politicians likely supported the plan favored by their major financial contributors.[62]

During the 1990s, the personal responsibility model for health continued to guide health policies. Health promotion efforts emphasized the importance of good choices in maintaining one's health. As part of the continued efforts to improve the health of Americans, the Institute of Medicine released in 1990 a follow-up report to *Healthy People*, which addressed new areas of concern, including mental health, health disparities among different social groups and childhood obesity.[63] Due to the significant increase in the number of overweight children in the 1980s and 1990s, the issue of childhood obesity had become a central issue in public health discussions.[64] Responsibility for improving the overall health of children was placed on schools and programs for children, parents, and the children themselves, who were encouraged to create healthy food choices for children and to increase children's activity levels to reduce risks of medical conditions associated with obesity.[65]

Legislation exemplified the continued overall focus on personal responsibility. In 1996, President Clinton approved the Personal Responsibility and

Work Opportunity Reconciliation Act, adding work requirements for welfare recipients, strengthening child support enforcement, and requiring minors with children to live in an adult-supervised environment to receive assistance.[66] Although President Clinton vetoed attempts to cut funds for health care, the emphasis on individual agency in other areas of welfare maintained the political focus on personal responsibility.

In the late 1990s, likely as a response to problems with managed care plans, the IOM reports on medical errors and subsequent improvements in the quality of patient care were released, alerting many people to the issue of patient safety. As mentioned earlier, the 1999 IOM report estimated that approximately 100,000 people die each year because of medical errors and that most errors occur because of flaws in the health care system.[67] The IOM report recommended developing national standards to improve patient safety and called for the American medical system to reduce medical errors by 50 percent within five years.[68] Two years later, in a follow-up report specifying the changes needed to improve patient safety, the IOM declared that the health care system needed to become more focused on patients and their safety.[69] Because of the IOM research, efforts to improve patient safety emerged in the late 1990s and continued into the 2000s. In 1997, the National Patient Safety Foundation (NPSF) founded to improve the quality of health care for patients by preventing patient injury, stated that "the system of health care is fallible and requires fundamental change" to improve patient safety.[70] And, to help develop effective strategies for improving patient safety, in 2001, Congress granted $50 million to the Agency of Healthcare Research and Quality to study the causes and prevention of medical errors.[71] To improve patient safety, consumers were advised to learn more about medical care so that they could protect themselves while in the hospital.[72] Consumers, then, were expected to not only take measures to maintain good health, but also were partially responsible for protecting their health while receiving medical treatment.

Overall, many concerns about individual health and health care reform were addressed in the 1990s. In this decade, attempts at universal health care failed, managed care plans were implemented nationwide, and publicity of the IOM reports and medical errors emphasized the issue of patient safety. At the same time, in the 1990s, expectations for personal responsibility expanded to include children. And the focus on the patient's role in reducing medical errors shifted some of the responsibility for quality medical treatment to the patient. These trends continued in the 2000s, with most Americans enrolled in managed care plans. Efforts to improve patient safety also continued through the implementation of patient safety standards, more quality control measures, and stricter regulations on medication labeling.[73]

In the 2000s, the rise in the publicity of medical errors, accompanied by increased problems with managed care and insurance, continued to weaken public confidence in medicine as an institution. Technology advances enabled people to seek medical advice beyond their primary physicians. With the growth of the Internet in the 1990s and into the twenty-first century, along with the advent of specialized health networks in television, many people increasingly researched their own health issues instead of relying solely on a medical professional's advice.[74] For example, *WebMD*, supported by the Mayo Clinic, allows consumers to research possible medical conditions for symptoms they were experiencing, along with treatment options.

Because of the problems in managed care plans and the publicity of medical errors, trust in the American health care system declined dramatically from the 1980s to the 2000s. In studying the Harris and NORC surveys of public trust in institutions, Pippa Norris noted that only 44 percent of Americans had a "great deal of confidence" in medicine in 2001, compared to 72 percent in 1966.[75] The publicity of scandals in the health care industry, such as cases of medical errors and stories about poor patient quality due to HMOs, hindered public trust in the health care industry.[76]

A lack of trust in the health care system can hinder the success of personal responsibility efforts. Dana Gelb Safran argued that the more people trust their physicians, the more likely they are to adapt healthy lifestyles that the physician recommends.[77] Blendon noted that while many people distrust the health care system, most still trust their primary physicians.[78] However, many people do not routinely visit the same physician and therefore may be less likely to heed their doctors' advice and adopt healthy lifestyles than those who regularly visit the same physician. Despite trust issues that may have hindered the success of personal responsibility efforts, politicians continued in the 2000s to emphasize the individual in maintaining good health. In 2000, a third IOM report highlighted health objectives for the American population to be achieved by the year 2010.[79]

Welfare reform during the first decade of the twenty-first century further emphasized the importance of individual behavior. In 2006, President Bush approved the Deficit Reduction Act, granting states more flexibility in devising and executing Medicaid programs. This plan aimed to "promote personal responsibility, independence, and choice."[80] For example, in West Virginia, members who received preventive health screenings, kept medical appointments, took prescribed medication, and followed other rules received additional medical care, unlimited prescriptions, and additional incentives like fitness-center memberships and healthy food vouchers.[81] While this plan may have theoretically promoted good health, it was pragmatically problematic. Robert Steinbrook explained that poor doctor-patient communication, problems with childcare or transportation, and other issues not addressed by the program, hindered many members' success in the program.[82] Gene Bishop and Amy Brodkey pointed out its flaws, stating, "This plan asks the most vulnerable population to do more with less ability to accomplish what we ask of them."[83] As with the personal behavior theory of disease causality in the 1830s, this program was not feasible for all Medicaid recipients and demonstrated significant flaws in the personal responsibility model as the primary guide for United States health policies. Despite these problems, however, based on the recent *Healthy People* report and legislation, the personal responsibility model continued to dominate in the 2000s.

FLAWED HEROES AND CARING CYNICS: "REALISTIC" PORTRAYALS OF HEALTH PROFESSIONALS

Medical dramas in the 1990s and early 2000s shifted from the paternalistic *Trapper John, M.D.*, and the cynical doctors in *St. Elsewhere*. The graphic nature, pace, and complex storylines of the programs *ER* and *Chicago Hope* (along with the British drama *Casualty*) broke ground in medical drama history.[84] Although these medical dramas used some traditional elements from the genre, such as a mix of serial and episodic plots, they presented the institution of medicine much more "realistically" than earlier dramas did.

As with the conventional medical drama formulas, *Chicago Hope* (1994–2000), *ER* (1994–2009), *House, M.D.* (2004–2012) and *Grey's Anatomy* (2005–present) portrayed health professionals as exceptional care providers, who are caring, compassionate, and so dedicated to patient care that they risk their careers and lives to save the patients. They repeatedly break hospital protocol to save patients. Dr. Doug Ross detoxes a heroin-addicted baby. Dr. Corday performs an illegal organ transplant to help an HIV-positive patient live longer. Dr. Izzie Stevens severs the cord of her patient's LVAD (a temporary heart device) to boost his position on the transplant list. And in nearly every episode of *House, M.D.*, Dr. House and his team violate hospital protocol to save their patients.

In contrast to earlier representations, these fictional professionals overcome many more personal and professional obstacles to treat patients. Dr. Aaron Schutt of *Chicago Hope* and *ER*'s Dr. Mark Greene successfully care for patients as they both battle brain cancer. Even with a Vicodin addiction, Dr. Gregory House is considered among the top in his field of diagnostics. Dr. Meredith Grey places her hand inside a man's chest, next to a highly unstable active bomb. Other health professionals in these four dramas face other obstacles, including mental illness, limb amputation, and violent assaults inside the hospital, as well as divorce, custody battles, and the deaths of loved ones. For the most part, even life-changing personal problems do not appear to distract the fictional health professionals, as they continue to demonstrate their exceptional skill.

Chicago Hope and *ER*, and later, *House, M.D.* and *Grey's Anatomy*, depicted health professionals as heroic but human in that they usually saved their patients but sometimes made mistakes. [85] From a content analysis of one season (1996–1997) of *Chicago Hope* and *ER*, Gregory Makoul and Limor Peer described the television physicians as sensitive professionals who behaved in an ethical manner. [86] Likewise, Cohen and Shafer, explained that the fictional health professionals in *ER* were "able to treat all comers with the most considerate of manners, rarely allowing external pressures to interfere with the instantly forged, yet remarkably intimate, doctor-patient relationship." [87] Vandekieft argued that medical dramas of the 1990s portrayed doctors as heroes "with human shortcomings," meaning that the fictional doctors went to great lengths to save their patients but sometimes failed or made mistakes. [88] And, as with earlier dramas, these shows largely ignored issues of health insurance and the cost of health care, regardless of how many expensive diagnostic tests or treatments were ordered. [89]

While most of the fictional characters were compassionate health professionals, a few were cynical and cantankerous, like Dr. Joseph Cacaci in *Chicago Hope* and Dr. Gregory House in *House, M.D.* To some viewers, the combination of these traits made the depictions of health professionals appear more "realistic" than in earlier programs. [90] Cohen and Shafer speculated that these idealistic yet realistic portrayals may have been popular because most people were disillusioned with the health care industry and therefore wanted to see positive images of physicians. [91] At the same time, savvy viewers wanted more realistic depictions than the infallible heroes of earlier dramas. [92] Like other television programs of the 1990s, these medical dramas featured much more diverse casts than those of any previous era. Not only were more women and people of color in the casts, but they also played doctors and other authoritative characters instead being in subordinate staff roles like nurses and orderlies. [93] In discussing *ER*'s appeal, George J. Annas described the medical professionals in the program as "young, good looking, ethnically diverse doctors and nurses" all of whom were romantically involved with each other. [94]

Unlike *St. Elsewhere*, producers of medical dramas of the 1990s and 2000s strived for authenticity by utilizing medical professionals in the creative process. As done for fictional medical programs of the past, medical professionals routinely reviewed scripts for accuracy, adding appropriate medical terminology to the dialogue. On sets, medical professionals helped actors understand "real-life" medicine. [95] The involvement of real-life health professionals demonstrated the commitment to medical accuracy, meaning, at least to some extent, that the health information conveyed to the viewing audience would be factual. For example, *ER* attempted to present accurate portrayals of patient care, illustrating the difficulty of correct diagnosis and effective treatment. [96]

Medical dramas of the 1990s and 2000s were also more realistic in that they featured a broader range of health professional roles than in earlier medical dramas, where the characters of nurses and other staff were minor in comparison to those of doctors.[97] Elka Jones argued that, especially in *ER*, nurses and paramedics played more central roles than in earlier programs.[98] However, some nursing professionals claimed the portrayals were still inadequate. Sandy and Harry Jacobs Summers noted that these programs showed doctors performing critical nursing tasks, downplaying the importance and power of nurses in providing patient care.[99] In 2005, the Center for Nursing Advocacy ranked *Grey's Anatomy*, *House, M.D.*, and *ER* as having three of the five worst portrayals of nursing for the year.[100] The advocacy group claimed that these programs depicted nurses as unimportant, barely visible, or working "as physicians' handmaidens."[101] Medical dramas like *ER* failed to address nursing shortages, which have been a growing problem in real-life hospitals.[102] Some have questioned the "realism" in the type of people who play health professionals in medical dramas. Alfred Peruzzi argued that *ER*, *House, M.D.*, and the medical comedy *Scrubs* misrepresent the medical profession by not including older health professionals or patients.[103] Other scholars have noted that health professionals in these programs were younger and more attractive than their real-life counterparts.[104]

Not all genres of television depicted health professionals so positively at this time. Chory-Assad and Tamborini found that, in comparison with television doctors in 1992 (the year of Pfau and colleagues' sample), television doctors "were often mean, unethical, incompetent, insubordinate, and sometimes criminal," identifying physician characters that used illegal drugs, murdered people and sold children on the black market[105] This sample included crime dramas, a genre that regularly features characters who are deviant and murderers, which likely explains why these findings vastly different from the positive portrayals noted by other scholars.

Despite some criticism and competing portrayals in other television genres, overall, medical dramas continued to be popular in the 1990s and 2000s. These programs offered depictions of health professionals that exemplified characteristics from several eras in television history. Medical dramas of the 1990s and 2000s, as an attempt at "realism," offered seemingly more complex depictions of health professionals. The next three chapters further explore the representations of health professionals and the medical profession in these contemporary dramas, examining how individual providers and patients are held responsible for good health and how these messages fit within changing public discourse about health care.

NOTES

Note: A portion of this chapter was based on the following book chapter: Foss, K. (2014). From Welby to McDreamy: What TV teaches us about doctors, patients, and the health care system (pp. 227–244). In D. Macey & K. M. Ryan (Eds.). *How Television Shapes Our Worldview: Media Representations of Social Trends and Change.* Lanham, MD. Lexington Books, 2014.

1. Burnham, "American Medicine's Golden Age: What Happened to It?"

2. Emanuel and Emanuel, "Four Models of the Physician-Patient Relationship"; Shore, *The Trust Crisis in Health Care.*

3. Arias, "United States Life Tables, 2008."

4. Ibid.

5. Tesh, *Hidden Arguments.*

6. Le Fanu, *The Rise and Fall of Modern Medicine.*

7. Ibid.

8. Ibid.

9. *Healthy People 2000: National Health Promotion and Disease Objectives.*

10. *Reducing Tobacco Use: A Report of the Surgeon General.*

11. Shore, *The Trust Crisis in Health Care.*

12. Millenson, "The Silence."

13. Ibid.

14. Ibid.

15. Health, *Healthy People.*

16. Ibid., 2-1.

17. Ibid.

18. Ibid., 2-8.

19. Le Fanu, *The Rise and Fall of Modern Medicine.*

20. Shore, *The Trust Crisis in Health Care.*

21. Laham, *A Lost Cause.*

22. Ibid.

23. Ibid.

24. Marmor, *Understanding Health Care Reform.*

25. Shore, *The Trust Crisis in Health Care.*

26. Ibid.

27. Wang, "Culture, Meaning and Disability"; Minkler, "Personal Responsibility for Health?"

28. Ibid.

29. Schulman, *The Seventies the Great Shift in American Culture, Society, and Politics.*

30. Irwin, "Reagan Stresses Family Values While Hart Laments Iran Scandal."

31. Bauer, Health Care Financial Management Association (U.S.), and Educational Foundation, *Not What the Doctor Ordered.*; Starr, *Remedy and Reaction.*

32. Shore, *The Trust Crisis in Health Care.*

33. Kirkwood and Brown, "Public Communication About the Causes of Disease"; Minkler, "Personal Responsibility for Health?"; Nurit Guttman, "On Being Responsible."

34. Allegrante and Green, "Sounding Board. When Health Policy Becomes Victim Blaming."

35. Ibid., 1528.

36. Ibid.

37. Chory-Assad and Tamborini, "Television Doctors."

38. Vandekieft, Gregg, "From City Hospital to ER: The Evolution of the Television Physician," 225.

39. Turow, *Playing Doctor*; Vandekieft, Gregg, "From City Hospital to ER: The Evolution of the Television Physician."

40. Turow, *Playing Doctor.*

41. Vandekieft, Gregg, "From City Hospital to ER: The Evolution of the Television Physician."

42. Ibid.

43. Turow, *Playing Doctor*.

44. Kletke et al., *The Demographics of Physician Supply*.

45. Ibid.

46. MacDonald, "Black Doctors on Television."

47. Ibid.

48. Engel, *Poor People's Medicine*; Bennfield, *Who Loses Coverage for How Long?*

49. Engel, *Poor People's Medicine*.

50. Ibid.

51. Laham, *A Lost Cause*.

52. Ibid.

53. Ibid.

54. Ibid.

55. Ibid.

56. Ibid.

57. Bauer, Health care Financial Management Association (U.S.), and Educational Foundation, *Not What the Doctor Ordered*; Zelman, *The Changing Health Care Marketplace*.

58. Bauer, Health Care Financial Management Association (U.S.), and Educational Foundation, *Not What the Doctor Ordered*.

59. Ibid.

60. Ibid.

61. Laham, *A Lost Cause*.

62. Ibid.

63. *Healthy People 2000: National Health Promotion and Disease Objectives.*

64. Berg, *Underage and Overweight*.

65. Ibid.

66. Kubiak, Siefert, and Boyd, "Empowerment and Public Policy."

67. America et al., *To Err Is Human*.

68. Ibid.

69. Spath, *Error Reduction in Health Care: A Systems Approach to Improving Patient Safety*.

70. "Mission and Vision | National Patient Safety Foundation."

71. *HHS Announces $50 Million Investment to Patient Safety*.

72. "20 Tips to Help Prevent Medical Errors."

73. Research, "Information for Consumers (Drugs) - Strategies to Reduce Medication Errors"; Nordenberg, "Make No Mistake! Medical Errors Can Be Deadly Serious."

74. Shore, *The Trust Crisis in Health Care*.

75. Norris, "Skeptical Patients: Performance, Social Capital, and Culture."

76. Blendon, "Why Americans Don't Trust the Government and Don't Trust Health Care."

77. Safran, "Patients' Trust in Their Doctors: Are We Losing Ground?".

78. Blendon, "Why Americans Don't Trust the Government and Don't Trust Health care."

79. America et al., *To Err Is Human*.

80. *The Deficit Reduction Act: Important Facts for State Government Officials*, 1.

81. Steinbrook, "Imposing Personal Responsibility for Health."

82. Ibid.

83. Bishop and Brodkey, "Personal Responsibility and Physician Responsibility — West Virginia's Medicaid Plan," 757.

84. Jacobs, *Body Trauma TV*.

85. Cohen and Shafer, "Images and Healers: A Visual History of Scientific Medicine."

86. Makoul and Peer, "Dissecting the Doctor Shows: A Content Analysis of ER and Chicago Hope."

87. Cohen and Shafer, "Images and Healers: A Visual History of Scientific Medicine," 211.

88. Vandekieft, Gregg, "From City Hospital to ER: The Evolution of the Television Physician."

89. Annas, "Sex, Money, and Bioethics Watching ER and Chicago Hope"; Turow, "Television Entertainment and the US Health-Care Debate."

90. Chory-Assad and Tamborini, "Television Doctors"; Jacobs, *Body Trauma TV*.

91. Cohen and Shafer, "Images and Healers: A Visual History of Scientific Medicine."

92. Ibid.

93. Jacobs, *Body Trauma TV*.

94. Annas, "Sex, Money, and Bioethics Watching ER and Chicago Hope," 40.

95. Jones, *ER*.

96. Ibid.

97. Turow, *Playing Doctor*; Kalisch and Kalisch, "A Comparative Analysis of Nurse and Physician Characters in the Entertainment Media."

98. Jones, "As Seen on TV."

99. Summers and Summers, "Viewpoint."

100. "Tarnished Images, plus a Few Gems."

101. Ibid., 33.

102. Summers and Summers, "Viewpoint."

103. Peruzzi, "View Askew. What Is Degrading the Teaching Hospital's Image?".

104. Chory-Assad and Tamborini, "Television Doctors"; Annas, "Sex, Money, and Bioethics Watching ER and Chicago Hope."

105. Chory-Assad and Tamborini, "Television Doctors," 514.

Chapter Four

"When we make mistakes, people die!" (Or do they?)

TV Medical Errors and the Code of Silence

Unlike the heroic doctors of television, real-life physicians and other types of health professionals frequently make mistakes. Most errors go unreported, or at least undisclosed, to the general public. This "code of silence," as it is called, is derived from the tradition of paternalistic medicine and high-regard for physicians, paired with a pervasive fear of malpractice litigation.[1] Indeed, one well-publicized lawsuit could destroy the career of a health care provider, even if the true culprit of the error was institutional, not individual.

The 1970s implementation of "informed consent," a trend toward patient participation, and the first comprehensive study on medical errors started shifting perceptions about restitution.[2] While the results of the medical error study were largely ignored in public discourse, heavy media coverage of tort reform and "frivolous lawsuits" heightened physicians' awareness of medical liability.[3] Thus, physicians deemed it necessary to purchase malpractice or liability insurance.[4] Since this time, malpractice insurance premiums have escalated, with surges in the 1970s, 1980s, and 1990s.[5]

How has the threat of malpractice impacted contemporary medicine? Besides encouraging health professionals to cover up medical mistakes, fears of malpractice liability have changed how many providers practice medicine. In the 1990s, the term "defensive medicine" was coined to describe how health professionals may modify their care in order to protect themselves against malpractice. The Office of Technology Assessment explains that defensive medicine occurs "when doctors order tests, procedures, or visits, or avoid certain high-risk patients or procedures, primarily (but not necessarily solely) because of concern about malpractice liability."[6] Defensive medicine can be through *assurance* behavior (ordering extra tests, being overly cautious in attending to patients, offering unneeded referrals to specialists) or *avoidance* behavior (avoiding patients or procedures perceived as risky or carrying high risk of complications).[7] A survey of physicians in high-risk specialties found that 93 percent of respondents admitted to practicing defensive medicine.[8] Furthermore, 43 percent of participants had taken preventive actions to reduce the possibility of malpractice, by omitting procedures with higher rates of complications and carefully screening patients to weed out those who appeared litigious or had complex medical conditions.[9] Yet, it is difficult to measure the extent to which this practice has negatively impacted medicine.[10]

News media have strongly contributed to the emphasis on individual medical errors, myths of abundant medical lawsuits (when in reality, most people do not sue), and stories of defensive medicine.[11] With the continuation of TV's heroic doctor, creators of entertainment media have taken a different approach. This chapter explores the responsibility of health professionals in *Chicago Hope*, *ER*, *House, M.D.*, and *Grey's Anatomy*, examining if and when these fictional providers make mistakes, the consequences (if any) for mistakes, and the extent to which institutional problems impact the quality of care. How do these programs negotiate the "heroic doctor," a staple role of television, when fears of litigation are causing real-life health professionals to doubt themselves?

Health professionals in these shows are nearly infallible, helping to treat and cure patients in even the most extreme situations. At the same time, unlike Marcus Welby and the other TV docs of an earlier era, health professional characters of the 1990s and 2000s sometimes made mistakes. In these medical dramas, cases of medical errors include delaying diagnosis or treatment, misdiagnosis, administering the wrong medicine or treatment, incorrectly performing a procedure, leaving surgical instruments inside a patient, or carrying out other actions differently than most competent health professionals would. Storylines indicate that a health professional is responsible when colleagues lectured the health professional, claiming that they would have administered a different medication or dosage, used a different procedure to treat the patient, taken a more thorough history, treated the patient's condition sooner, taken a better look at the results of diagnostic tests or performed other actions. Health professionals face various consequences for their mistakes in the shows.

ERRORS MAKE HEALTH PROFESSIONALS BETTER PROVIDERS

In the four dramas, medical errors cause health professionals to become better health care providers, improving the overall quality of care. No errors due to inexperience occurred in *Chicago Hope, House, M.D.*, or *Grey's Anatomy* (despite the numerous surgical interns in the show). Yet, in *ER*, medical students, interns, and residents unsuccessfully attempted procedures without the proper training and supervision, causing harm to their patients. They learn from their mistakes and eventually become excellent physicians.

Throughout season one of *ER*, medical students John Carter and Deb Chen (also referred to as Jing Mei) compete for cases in order to expand their portfolios of procedures completed. In "House of Cards,"[12] Carter, guided by a senior resident, learns how to put a central line into a man's chest. Chen sees Carter doing this procedure and exclaims, "You're doing a central line?" In the next scene, Chen and a nursing student, Wendy, have trouble inserting an IV in a patient. Wendy suggests that the patient needs a central line and leaves to find a more experienced health professional. When Wendy returns, she sees Chen inserting the central line. Wendy says, "Are you crazy? You're not allowed to do a central line." Chen responds, "I was just going to get it started but then it seemed so easy." Chen pulls a tool out from the chest and assures Wendy, "It's fine. Look." But Chen quickly starts to panic, asking, "Where's the guide wire?" The camera shot cuts to surgical resident Dr. Peter Benton declaring that the man needs emergency surgery. Chen flees the room and soon thereafter withdraws from medical training at Cook County General Hospital. Five seasons of *ER* later, Chen returns and tells others that her parents bought her way into another program. As evidence that Chen's medical skills had dramatically improved while she was gone, she is chosen as Chief Resident and successfully treats many patients.

In season three of *ER*, Dr. Peter Benton, a skilled surgical resident, does a pediatric surgery rotation under the supervision of renowned pediatric surgeon, Dr. Abby Keaton. Benton's selfishness and overconfidence in his surgical skill become problematic in his first unsupervised attempt at pediatric surgery. In "Fear of Flying,"[13] Keaton and Benton operate on an infant with abdominal injuries. As they are about to close the wound, Keaton asks Benton to finish, instructing him not to do additional procedures. After Keaton leaves, Benton scrapes the infant's liver with a scalpel, causing it to bleed profusely. Instead of paging Keaton, Benton attempts to stitch up the liver, resulting in massive blood loss for the fragile patient. Finally, Keaton is called in. She works frantically to keep the baby alive. Once she stabilizes the infant, Keaton confronts Benton, telling him, "You didn't know what the hell you were doing. The second you realized you had screwed up, you should have called me. Why did I find three stitches in there?" Keaton continues, "Because you blindly and arrogantly think that you have all the answers. If that baby dies, it'll be my responsibility, but it will be your fault." At the end of this episode, close-up shots of the delicate infant emphasize the gravity of Benton's mistake. Wrapped in gauze, the tiny baby lies still as her blood circulates through the bypass machine and back into her fragile form. The baby slowly recovers and her parents are never informed of the mistake. Benton does not permanently enter pediatrics, but repeatedly proves his exceptional talent as a general surgeon throughout the next four seasons of *ER*. For example, in season five, on the scene of a boating accident, Benton demonstrates his outstanding abilities when he saves a man using only saran wrap and a fishing lure.

Nurse and medical student Abby Lockhart makes a mistake due to inexperience in season six of *ER*. In "Under Control,"[14] Lockhart and Dr. Chen insert a drainage tube in the abdominal cavity of an older African American man with terminal colon cancer. After Chen leaves the room, Lockhart attempts to adjust the tube by herself. The patient moans in pain. Later, surgeon Peter Benton informs the patient he needs surgery to repair his perforated diaphragm (from the tube), calling Lockhart's mistake a "known complication of the procedure." The patient refuses the operation because of his terminal cancer. In private, Lockhart says to Benton, "He's going to die because I made a mistake." Benton responds, "He's going to die anyway." Lockhart's supervisor, Dr. Greene, determines that Lockhart provided an incomplete medical history to Dr. Chen, which meant that the procedure was performed incorrectly. Dr. Chen faces no consequences and Greene advises Lockhart to practice procedures in the pathology lab. At the end of the episode, Lockhart practices on a cadaver—her former patient.

In comparison to seasons one through nine of *ER*, in seasons ten and eleven, most of the main characters are medical students or junior medical residents. These inexperienced characters often misdiagnose patients or attempt unsupervised procedures. In "Shifts Happen,"[15] staffing shortages for the night shift leave only one attending physician on duty. Second-year resident Dr. Greg Pratt treats numerous patients, including a boy with a quarter lodged in his throat. Because of a lengthy delay for the gastrointestinal specialist (after fourteen hours in the E.R. waiting room), Pratt retrieves the quarter himself, using an inflated tube in the boy's throat. Smiling, Pratt gives the quarter to the boy's parents, saying, "Here. One for the piggy bank." Later, the boy starts vomiting blood. Upon examining the boy, surgeon Elizabeth Corday determines that Pratt tore the boy's esophagus with the tube and tells him, "You know, you're lucky this happened while they were still here, otherwise this boy could be dead." Besides Corday's verbal reprimand of Pratt, he faces no other consequences.

In other episodes of these two seasons, medical student Neela Rasgotra, and emergency medicine residents Michael Gallant, Ray Barnett and Archie Morris were depicted as making errors in diagnosis and treatment. Other than a reprimand from their supervisors, these professionals face no consequences for mistakes. Because they learn from their mistakes, becoming skilled health care providers, these health professionals were depicted only as inexperienced and not as grossly incompetent.

In *ER* and *House, M.D.*, health professionals also commit errors when they were temporarily distracted by personal problems. In season six of *ER*, a patient stabs Dr. John Carter in the kidneys with a butcher knife. During his long recovery, Carter becomes addicted to narcotics, an addiction that begins to interfere with his ability to treat patients. In the episode "Such Sweet Sorrow,"[16] Carter administers an antibiotic to a patient with known sulfa allergies, causing anaphylaxis. He panics and rips out her IV. Another doctor witnesses Carter lie to a nurse about the IV and order some Benadryl for the reaction. Carter then runs to the bathroom, sits on the toilet, and sobs.

Although the patient recovers, this mistake and Carter's other erratic behavior prompt an intervention in the next episode, "May Day." Carter denies his addiction to the other health professionals:

> Carter: Can anybody tell me that uh, uh that I have endangered patients? I mean can anybody here say that my performance has changed? Hmm? That I'm some kind of a liability?
> Chen: John, you put a patient into anaphylactic shock by giving her Bactrim when she told you that she was allergic to it.

The doctors ultimately convince Carter to admit himself to a drug rehabilitation center. When Carter returns in the next season, he is no longer using narcotics and is again a skilled physician. Carter demonstrates his skill in "The Crossing,"[17] when he successfully performs a double amputation on a man trapped under a train, despite limited surgical training, poor lighting, and the difficulty of performing surgery in the field.

In the *ER* episode "The Visit,"[18] surgeon Dr. Elizabeth Corday's eagerness to leave work results in a patient's paralysis. Throughout this episode, Corday and her fiancé Dr. Mark Greene anxiously tell other doctors of their vacation plans following their shifts. Toward the end of her shift, Corday diagnoses a middle-aged surfer, Al Patterson, with a herniated disc. Corday recommends endoscopic surgery to repair the injury and tells the patient that the procedure will only take an hour and will only involve "a couple of stitches and a Band-Aid." Later, Chief of Staff Dr. Robert Romano interrupts another case to question Corday's decision to use endoscopy to repair Patterson's disc. As Corday justifies her decision, Romano adds, "And you can still ditch out of here for your romantic weekend." Corday angrily replies, "What the hell are you insinuating? That I chose an inappropriate course of surgery to accommodate my weekend plans?" Following this interaction, however,

Corday promises Greene that she will finish by 6:00 and asks a nurse to inform her of the time during the surgery.

As Corday performs the endoscopic procedure, the image of the patient's spinal cord appears on a screen. Corday remarks on blood that oozed around the spinal cord, which is visible on the screen, and cauterizes the bleed. At this point, clear liquid pools on top of the spinal cord. The anesthesiologist tells Corday, "Uh, we got some leaking fluid." Corday responds, "It's just irrigation solution. It's looking good." She reassures the patient (who is awake), "You'll be hanging ten before you know it."

After Corday leaves for the weekend, the patient complains of severe back pain. When Romano asks him to roll onto his side, the patient tries but cannot move his lower body. Romano touches the patient's leg, asking, "Can you feel this?" Romano and the nurses roll the patient, which reveals soaked bandages covering his back. Romano says, "Mr. Patterson, you're leaking spinal fluid. It's probably a cord compression. Let's get him to the OR. Find me Elizabeth Corday." Due to Corday's negligence, the patient is permanently paralyzed.

Dr. Corday is sued for negligence after her actions led to a patient's paralysis. During the deposition, Corday publicly denies the accusations that her ability was impaired. However, she privately admits to Dr. Greene that she made a mistake, demonstrating her sense of guilt about her actions.

> Corday: I lied. I lied. The fact is I rushed. I rushed through and didn't inspect the entire surgical field. That man will never walk again because I wanted to get out early for the weekend and I couldn't even claim responsibility. I sat there and I swore to God and I lied to save myself.

Several episodes later, the error is ultimately attributed to a product recall of one of the surgical instruments. Corday faces no disciplinary actions and the lawsuit is settled. Yet even though Corday briefly questions her surgical skill following her error, a subsequent episode, titled "Surrender," portrays her exceptional abilities in a similar spinal cord operation that she successfully performs.

Dr. Robert Chase in *House, M.D.* makes a critical error when he is distracted by the news of his father's death. The episode, aptly entitled "The Mistake,"[19] unfolds through flashbacks prompted by conversations with the hospital's attorney, Stacy Warner. In this episode, Chase learns that his father died of lung cancer. As he hangs up the phone, a patient enters the room for a follow-up visit and mentions that her stomach pain has not subsided. At this point, according to the other doctors, Chase should have asked about other symptoms, which would have indicated a more serious problem. Instead, Chase prescribes some antacids and sends the woman home. A few hours later, paramedics bring the woman into the hospital. After the other physicians determine the patient has bleeding ulcers and a perforation in her stomach, Dr. House confronts Chase about his actions. Chase tells House that she was "fine" a few hours before. House responds:

> House: She was not fine two hours ago. Did she mention stomach pain?
> Chase: Yeah, so I gave her a stronger—
> House: You didn't do an exam?
> Chase: She just came in for a follow-up. The results of the pathergy test.
> House: Did you listen to her stomach? Check her vitals?
> Chase: Maybe if she'd said something about taking ibuprofen, mentioned the rectal bleeding—
> House (interrupts): Yeah! Why didn't she go to med school like you did? Diarrhea, blood in the stool, these are routine questions!
> Chase: That doctors skip all the time. It was a minor mistake. I couldn't have known this was gonna happen.
> House: Mistakes are as serious as the results they cause! This woman could die because you were too lazy to ask one simple question!

Because of the perforation, the patient's stomach acid causes a serious infection, damaging her liver. The patient's brother lies about his Hepatitis C and donates part of his liver. Two months later, the woman develops cancer in the diseased liver and dies. Chase's medical error occurred because of his grief, not overall incompetence. He faces a brief suspension and the mistake is noted in his file. Yet, no lawsuit is filed and the error actually improves Chase's abilities as a care provider. Later storylines convey that Chase has become more assertive and protective of his patients, as illustrated in "Finding Judas," when he saves a little girl from unnecessary amputation.

Contrary to news media, which have framed errors as the product of inept doctors, only three truly incompetent fictional health professionals appear in the 536 episodes studied. These characters are not regular characters, but limited to the storylines about their negligent behavior. For example, in *Chicago Hope*, a lab technician failed to notify hospital administrators of a case of drug-resistant tuberculosis, exposing all emergency room patients to the disease. The technician was fired for his error. A more extensive case appears in "Fear of Flying" in *ER*, after paramedics bring a football player with a severed foot to the hospital.[20] A nurse named Rhonda is asked to prepare the foot in ice for reattachment surgery. She becomes confused and ices the football instead, placing the severed foot next to the patient's belongings. Once the mistake is discovered, nursing supervisor Carol Hathaway says to Rhonda, "It was the most incompetent horrifying thing I've ever seen. And because you didn't ice the foot, they can't reattach it." Rhonda attributes her mistake to hospital administration (floating her to areas in which she has no experience) and quits her job. Yet Rhonda's carelessness, as reinforced by Hathaway's comments, conveyed that Rhonda was not qualified to adequately treat patients. Rhonda does not appear in subsequent episodes, suggesting that inept professionals are quickly dismissed, thus protecting the overall quality of care.

In the *Grey's Anatomy* episode "The Self-Destruct Button,"[21] anesthesiologist Dr. Taylor is caught performing surgery while intoxicated. After Taylor denies the alcohol on his breath, Intern George O'Malley pleads, "There is a two-year-old girl on this table. You shouldn't take advantage of someone else's vulnerability." Neurosurgeon Dr. Derek Shepherd dismisses O'Malley, as Taylor administers the anesthesia. In the middle of the surgery, the little girl begins to wake up, indicating Taylor's negligence. Afterward, Shepherd praises O'Malley for his actions, saying, "I was out of line. Somebody should have taken responsibility." Shepherd continues, "It should have been me. You didn't deserve what happened to you today. You did the right thing, code or no code." Overall, the patient is not permanently harmed, and the incompetent anesthesiologist is no longer depicted as practicing medicine. In these cases, the primary physician characters fired the incompetent health professionals, thus demonstrating their integrity and skill as health professionals and their impact in improving the overall quality of care.

HEALTH PROFESSIONALS ARE AT FAULT FOR ERRORS CAUSED BY THE HEALTH CARE SYSTEM

Health professionals are portrayed as skilled and competent people who made mistakes because of problems with the health care system. These characters are often shown working shifts longer than 12 hours. Such exhaustion caused several fatal mistakes. *Chicago Hope*'s cardiothoracic surgeon Dr. Kate Austin makes a critical error that leads to a patient's death in "The Ethics of Hope."[22] As the episode begins, Austin is operating on a patient when she asks surgeon Dr. Billy Kronk, "Hey Billy, Do you mind closing for me? I've been on 16 straight hours." Kronk agrees and finishes the operation. The patient is moved to the recovery room, where she goes into cardiac arrest and dies.

During the Morbidity & Mortality (M&M) conference, Austin learns that Kronk had clamped a damaged vessel in the patient's heart when the patient was first brought to the emergency room. Austin never removed the clamp or repaired the vessel. Another doctor in the meeting speculates that, after surgery, the clamp shifted, causing the patient to bleed to death. An X-ray is made of the patient's chest and delivered to Austin's office. A close-up of the X-ray shows a large clamp across the patient's rib cage. Later, when Kronk examines the X-ray, he comments, "If a jury ever saw that . . . It looks huge." Yet, all parties involve discourage Austin or others from informing the patient's family. Chief of Staff Dr. Phillip Watters ends the M & M conference with, "A reminder to all that nothing said here gets out. This is a sealed proceeding." Later, the hospital's legal counsel warns Austin not to inform the patient's family.

> Austin: Their daughter is dead. Are you telling me we're supposed to cover it up?
> Legal Counsel: They are free to look at all the operation reports. They can hire a lawyer.
> Austin: But they're not going to do that. They don't have a hint that anything is wrong. They're prepared to bury their daughter tomorrow along with the evidence.
> Legal: That's the way it goes sometimes.

This conversation not only discourages disclosure, but the legal counsel's statements imply that it is the responsibility of the patient's family to investigate her case to determine if an error occurred. Austin's colleague neurosurgeon Dr. Schutt makes a similar argument—that disclosure could hinder doctors from freely discussing medical mistakes, stating, "You would be undermining the only mechanism we have for making sure the same thing didn't happen twice." Austin decides not to inform the patient's family. However, years later, Austin's guilt over the error prompts her to inform the family that the error occurred. Because Austin is not affiliated with the hospital when she discloses the error, she faces no disciplinary actions for her mistake. Austin makes no further mistakes in other episodes, wins an award for her skill and is elected chief of surgery.

Fatigue also leads to a medical error for surgical intern Dr. Meredith Grey in "Shake Your Groove Thing"[23] of *Grey's Anatomy*. Prior to the surgery, Grey speaks of her exhaustion: "Look, I haven't slept in 48 hours. I'm getting my first shot at heart surgery this morning." During the operation, Grey is holding the patient's heart in her hand as she closes her eyes for a moment. As she jerks awake, she moves her hand, squeezing the patient's heart. Cardiothoracic surgeon Preston Burke asks, "What was that, Dr. Grey?" She replies, "Sorry, it slipped. My hands." The surgeons get the patient's heart beating and close the wound. Later, an interaction between Grey and intern Dr. O'Malley suggests that Grey believed she made a mistake.

> Grey: I think maybe I did something to the heart when I was holding it. I nodded off a little. Squeezed it.
> O'Malley: Oh, please. The heart's a tough muscle. It could take a squeeze or two.
> Grey: My fingernail popped the glove. Cut straight through. George, what if I punctured Mrs. Patterson's heart?
> O'Malley: If. . . . If you had punctured it, you would have known when they reperfused. They got her heart beating. The woman's okay.

Following surgery, the patient's heart stops beating and she dies, which Dr. Burke attributes to congenitally thin cardiac walls. Yet, Grey blames herself and informs the family and hospital attorney of her actions, resulting in one-month probation. Despite the admission of the error, it is not apparent that a lawsuit was filed.

Hospital staffing shortages also cause individual medical errors in *ER*. In the episode, "Post Mortem"[24] the nurses hold a "sick-out," in which the ER nurses call in sick to make a statement to hospital management about their union goals. Nurse manager Carol Hathaway is the only regular nurse working alongside a group of temporary nurses, who are clearly unaware of ER procedures and protocol. One patient, a homeless African American man, dies in the trauma room. During clean-up, Hathaway discovers that she administered the wrong typed-blood to the dead patient (A-positive instead of O-negative). Hathaway reports her error to Dr. Kerry Weaver, the acting Chief of Emergency Medicine. Instead of reprimanding Hathaway for the fatal error, Dr. Weaver sympathizes with her, stating, "It was an honest mistake. You were the only RN in the room. We were all filling roles we weren't accustomed to." Hathaway responds, "It still doesn't take away the basic error. I did not check the label." Against Weaver's advice, Hathaway reports her error to hospital administrators, who use Hathaway's error as ammunition against the nurses, blaming their absence for creating an environment that led to her mistake. Eventually, the administration suspends Hathaway, which appears to have greater ramifications for the nurses than her initial mistake did. In Hathaway's absence, a number of mishaps occur, including a flood of too many supplies, suggesting that for the ER, Hathaway's self-induced punishment is worse than her fatal mistake. And, during her suspension, Hathaway demonstrates exceptional skill as a nurse when she saves a robbery victim by using a tampon applicator to create a tracheotomy.

The set-up of the emergency room triage also contributes to medical errors. As with the patient who had swallowed the quarter, in *ER*, patients waited a long time to receive medical attention, resulting in serious consequences. For example, in "Out of Africa,"[25] an overweight African American woman collapses and dies after sitting in the waiting room all day. The doctors determine that massive bleeding in her brain caused her death. Dr. Luca Kovac tells a resident that the woman's death could have been prevented:

> Kovac: A five-minute physical exam could have picked up the bleed. We would have had time to operate. Instead, she waited 11 hours and left without being seen. This woman had nowhere else to go. If we can't find a way to take care of people like her, nobody will.

This case suggested that the faulty design of the fictional emergency room system caused delayed treatment for patients. Indeed, real-life studies have demonstrated that ER waiting times increase the likelihood of complications and other adverse events.[26] The absence of errors from most episodes despite these difficult working conditions demonstrated the exceptional skill of the fictional health professionals.

CONSEQUENCES FOR HEALTH PROFESSIONALS DEPEND ON PATIENT ADVOCACY AND DISCLOSURE

When fictional health professionals are depicted as responsible for medical errors, they face consequences ranging from minimal, such as a private reprimand, to severe, which includes lawsuits or disciplinary action. The severity of the consequences for health professionals depends on the medical outcome for the patient, the extent to which the patients and their families were informed of the error, and the amount of support that the patient had.

In many cases, consequences are minimal, limited to private lectures from a colleague or supervisor, as evident in Lockhart's accidental diaphragm perforation and Pratt's torn esophagus. They do not face formal reviews or other consequences, despite the severity of the injuries from the mistakes. Such minor consequences correlated with the lack of error disclosure. In all four of dramas, other health professionals, hospital administrators, and attorneys strongly discouraged informing patients and their families of medical errors to patients or their families, with the rationale that nondisclosure protected 1) other doctors at the hospital, encouraging them to discuss cases among themselves in order to prevent errors from reoccurring; 2) health professionals' careers so that they could continue to save lives; 3) patient's families from experiencing more grief in knowing that their loved one's suffering could have been prevented.

These arguments reflect rationale that some health professionals have used for nondisclosure of medical errors. Research published in 2012 found that many physicians admit to some dishonesty with their patients.[27] One-third of the doctors surveyed did not believe that serious medical errors should be disclosed to patients.[28] Other scholars have noted such resistance to error disclosure, even with alarmingly high rates of medical mistakes.[29] Instead, many physicians favor self-policing over institutional change—a tradition which has created a climate for errors.[30] Again, this lack of disclosure has meant that most people do not file malpractice lawsuits, even with legitimate claims, because they are unaware that negligence has occurred, which only reinforces a flawed system that breeds errors.[31]

The extent to which fictional patients had emotional support influenced the severity of the consequences for erring health professionals. With the exception of the paralyzed surfer, all patients who received financial restitution had family members supporting them, demonstrating the importance of patient advocacy and shifting blame to the families. Fictional patients who were homeless were especially treated poorly, as evident by the patient given the wrong blood type, whose death was initially dismissed. Real-life studies on the experiences of homeless people with health care providers have shown that they often feel discriminated against, stigmatized, and unwanted. [32] These patients have also reported feeling "invisible" and less important than other patients. [33] Such perceptions have significant implications. Homeless people are three times more likely to visit the ER in a year than the general population because many lack access to regular providers and have greater incidence of the need for care, due to mental illness and chronic disease. [34] Therefore, negative experiences discourage homeless people from seeking care, even when they need it the most. [35] Overall then, TV's representations that connect consequences to advocacy reflect and perpetuate real-life messages about patient hierarchy, without calling attention to the problems of this practice.

HEALTH PROFESSIONALS CAN'T HELP PATIENTS WHO DON'T HELP THEMSELVES

The fictional health professionals are depicted as not responsible for medical errors with irresponsible patients. Some episodes focus more on the patient's poor life choices than on the health professional's mistake. When health professionals make mistakes while treating smokers, drug users, or homeless people, the patients were culpable for initially causing their ill health. For example, in the *Chicago Hope* episode "Lamb to the Slaughter,"[36] the health professionals fail to clamp a major artery in the heart of an African American male gang member who had been shot. Although this action causes the patient's death, no investigation is conducted.

And in the "Histories" episode of *House, M.D.*, Dr. Eric Foreman dismisses a homeless woman because he believes that she is faking her symptoms. Foreman tells another doctor, Dr. Wilson, "She doesn't want to be discharged. She's manipulating me." He speculates that the patient overdosed on insulin, explaining to Wilson: "Look, a seizure buys her a place to sleep while the nice doctors run their tests, maybe a few free meals." Due to Wilson's and House's insistence, the patient is not discharged. Because of Foreman's doubt in the patient's complaints, he misses environmental factors that could cause illness—particularly the bats in her cardboard box house, as well as her physical symptoms of light sensitivity and erratic behavior. House, not Foreman, diagnoses the patient with rabies, which had become too advanced to be treated. Foreman's delayed diagnosis leads to the patient's death. Yet, the patient's squalid living conditions appear to excuse Foreman for missing the patient's diagnosis.

In season three of *House, M.D.*, Dr. Foreman once again misjudges a patient, leading to delayed diagnosis. In "House Training,"[37] Lupe, a twenty-eight-year-old woman of color, lives "in the projects" and had experienced many periods of unemployment. After meeting the patient, Foreman calls her a "drug-using scam artist," even though Lupe insists that she is clean. Foreman lectures Lupe on her choices, telling her, "You make bad decisions every day of your life. Stop doing drugs. Stop having fun. Go back to school and get your G.E.D." Foreman focuses more on reprimanding her for her life choices than examining her, as he quickly decides she has cancer. He treats Lupe with radiation, destroying her immune system. After the radiation, the diagnostics team determines that the patient has an infection. Unfortunately, the doctors determine that an infection is actually making her ill, which her body cannot fight because of the radiation. After the patient dies, Foreman admits his error to his supervisor, Dr. House, stating, "I killed her." House downplays Foreman's mistake, reminding him of the patients they do save. Here, the emphasis on the patient's unhealthy lifestyle, combined with the lack of consequences for the fatal mistake, implicate Lupe, not the physicians, for her death.

Storylines also convey that patients who endanger their own health by using substances were responsible when the outcome of treatments was adverse. In the third and fourth seasons of *ER*, Dr. Greene misses the pregnancy of African American woman who uses crack. In "When the Bough Breaks,"[38] Nurse Hathaway follows a trail of blood into the women's restroom, where the patient is in labor and soon delivers a stillborn baby. After reviewing the woman's charts, Hathaway tells Dr. Greene, who had treated the woman multiple times, that he missed her pregnancy. He becomes angry, replying, "What could we have done? We can't help people who can't help themselves." She responds, "Those are exactly the people that we should be helping." But she does not report the mistake to the patient or hospital administration, suggesting that because the patient's crack usage likely caused the stillbirth, even if Greene had caught the pregnancy early, he could not have saved the baby.

Medical errors that occur to heavy smokers are also dismissed. In "Shake Your Groove Thing"[39] in *Grey's Anatomy*, surgeons notice a white mass on the lungs of a heavy smoker. The Chief of Surgery Richard Webber tells Intern Dr. O'Malley to prepare the patient for surgery and says, "Says here we operated on her back in '99, so Mrs. Drake has been through this before, but talk her through it anyway. And resist the anti-smoking lecture, she feels bad enough already." As Webber leaves the room, O'Malley asks another surgeon about the potential impact of the X-ray of the cancerous lungs, saying, "So you think if they put a picture of these next to a pack of cigarettes, people would stop smoking?" Bailey shakes her head. Later, as O'Malley preps the patient, Mrs. Drake, she complains of chronic pain.

> Mrs. Drake: The surgery before was supposed to help, but it...it never felt right.
> O'Malley: Probably would have been a good idea to quit smoking.
> Mrs. Drake: I did! Four pack a day habit. Oh, it was hell.
> The nurse enters and gives Mrs. Drake a blanket as she and O'Malley continue talking.
> Mrs. Drake: It didn't do any damn good.
> O'Malley: Really? Because it looked, I mean, from the damage, we all thought you probably were still smoking.
> Mrs. Drake: Cold turkey. Five years ago. What do I get for my trouble? I still had to quit my job at the restaurant. But even sitting, it hurt.

During the operation, the doctors discover a surgical towel inside the woman's chest. As the towel is lifted out of the patient, O'Malley asks, "Where did that come from?" Cardiothoracic surgeon Dr. Preston Burke replies, "Best guess, her surgery five years ago." At this point, Bailey states, "Something careless this way comes." They deduce that Burke left the towel inside the patient in her previous surgery. When he informs the patient, she does not become angry or blame Burke; nor does she file suit against the hospital, even though the towel had caused her pain since the initial surgery. In fact, the woman simply expresses relief that her pain had "not just been in her mind." The emphasis on the woman's poor health habits (smoking) combined with the lack of consequences for Dr. Burke imply that because she brought her need for the first surgery upon herself, the woman, not Burke, is responsible for her pain, even though he made the mistake.

In season 11 of *ER*, (former nurse and now intern) Dr. Lockhart's patient, a former heavy smoker with emphysema, goes into cardiac arrest because Lockhart was not monitoring him properly. The attending physician calls the error a "classic intern mistake." Yet, despite the acknowledgement of the error, Lockhart faces no consequences for her actions. Another doctor tells Lockhart, "The guy is fine. It's not your fault he smoked two packs a day for decades." The lack of consequences, combined with the emphasis on the patient's poor health choices, depicted the patient as responsible for his health, even when a doctor makes mistakes in his health care.

Many fictional patients in *House, M.D.* experience ill effects from a wrong diagnosis or treatment because they are not forthcoming about their past. In the pilot episode, Dr. House explains that he does not trust patients because, "Everybody lies." This statement is well-supported throughout the program. In "Daddy's Boy,"[40] for example, a boy's treatment is delayed due to his father's dishonesty. The father, Mr. Hall, initially tells House and the diagnostics team that he owns a construction company. When House learns that Mr. Hall actually manages a salvage yard, he confronts the man.

> House: You lied.
> Mr. Hall: What are you talking about?
> House: Oh, yeah, of course in this family, you probably need more specifics. You told us you owned a construction company, not a salvage yard.
> Mr. Hall: I know the way things work. The better my job, the better my son gets treated.
> House: Right, that's why I'm mad. We wasted all that filet mignon on you.

The doctors determine that an object from the salvage yard that Mr. Hall gave to his son is radioactive, which has caused radiation poisoning and a tumor on the patient's spinal column. After surgery, the patient develops an infection, which his body cannot fight because the radiation destroyed his immune system. The doctors inform Mr. Hall that his son will likely die. Since Mr. Hall's son is diagnosed immediately after House learns the truth, this episode conveys that Hall's dishonesty led to delayed treatment of his son, constructing Mr. Hall, not the doctors, as responsible for the son's death.

In "Humpty Dumpty,"[41] a patient's lie about his occupation costs him his right hand. The patient, named Alfredo, works as a handyman during the day for Dr. Lisa Cuddy and works a second job as a janitor at night. Alfredo is admitted to the hospital with trouble breathing and poor circulation. The diagnostics team misdiagnoses Alfredo first with a clotting problem and then with pneumonia. His condition continues to worsen as his hand blackens and becomes gangrenous, forcing doctors to amputate. After the hand is removed, Dr. Chase notices that fingers on the other hand have begun to darken and that the patient's organs are failing. At this point, House confronts the patient about his suspicions about his second job, asking him, "What were you going to do tonight? What job do you have on Saturday nights?" At a nearby warehouse, the diagnostics team finds Alfredo's brother handling chickens at a cockfight. Alfredo is then successfully treated for his psittacosis (a disease contracted from chickens) and his remaining hand heals. House's quick diagnosis and treatment after he learns the truth suggests that had Alfredo been forthcoming, he would have kept the use of his hand. The final shot of the episode emphasizes the consequences for Alfredo as he gazes at his bandaged stump. Since Alfredo's dishonesty causes the delay in treatment, he is depicted as responsible for the medical outcome, in this case, the amputation of his hand.

Numerous other examples exist in *House, M.D.*, justifying actions that would otherwise be called mistakes. For example, in "Fidelity,"[42] a woman lies about promiscuity, causing her to undergo unnecessary painful treatments and to lapse into a coma from a delay in treating the disease before she is cured. The patient's dishonesty about her sexual history depicts her, not the doctors, as responsible for the unnecessary treatment and delay in diagnosis. Likewise, when a farmer lies about a bite on his leg in "Three Stories,"[43] the doctors' treatment causes analphylaxis and delays treating the damaged tissue. The final scene shows the man back on his farm lifting up his pants to adjust his prosthetic leg. In these cases, health professionals are not depicted as responsible when their actions cause negative medical outcomes for the patient. These cases convey that when patients fail to practice healthy behaviors or provide accurate information to health professionals, then the treating professional is less responsible when problems arose. The devastating consequences shown for many of the fictional patients emphasizes the gravity of their decisions and behaviors.

CONCLUSION

Medical dramas generally construct health professionals as heroes who risked their lives to save patients. At an individual level, cases of medical error were shown as making main characters better at treating patients or by leading to the dismissal of incompetent ones. At the institutional level, however, little change was noted, even when it was portrayed that flaws in the health care system contribute to errors. The abilities of these professionals to overcome obstacles created by a flawed health care system mask problems in the fictional health care system that likely translate to real life. The lack of medical mistakes in the four dramas may bring up questions of accuracy in medical dramas—a theme that has been present since the 1950s.[44] From a cultivation perspective, these idealistic depictions may be problematic in that they may reinforce perceptions that medical errors are rare and are limited to a few individuals, instead of highlighting the institutional flaws that cause most medical mistakes.[45]

The rarity of medical errors presented in the medical dramas coincides with what scholars have reported as general trends, overall, in popular media, which may help explain why many people underestimate errors in real life.[46] However, in contrast to the rare depictions of errors in the dramas studied here, these scholars stated that popular media report errors as the result of incompetent physicians. Although a few cases of errors due to incompetence were noted, most portrayals of medical mistakes in the dramas helped health professionals become exceptional care providers by learning from their mistakes, meaning that the fictional health care system is untouched.

When health professionals were depicted as making mistakes, consequences for their mistakes largely depended on patient advocacy. Hospital administrators and fellow physicians discouraged each other from informing patients and their families of mistakes, thus reinforcing a "code of silence." Reasons for not disclosing the errors were, ostensibly, to protect the quality of patient care. In real life, doctors have used similar arguments to uphold the code of silence, including the contention that patients benefit from nondisclosure.[47] And despite real-life trends toward defensive medicine, this practice is not addressed in the medical dramas. This absence may be explained by the rarity of medical errors in the programs and the lack of insurance and policy discussions overall. The four dramas showed that fictional patients without a network of support rarely received restitution for medical errors. Thus, these cases suggest that patients who lack family or friends in the real-world health system may be less likely to receive restitution for medical errors. In summary, contemporary TV producers mostly uphold and protect the heroic doctor, with occasional errors that only reinforce the overall quality of care provided by the hospitals.

NOTES

Note: A portion of this chapter first appeared as the following article: Foss, K. (2011). "When we make mistakes, people die!" Constructions of responsibility for medical errors in televised medical dramas, 1994-2007. *Communication Quarterly*, 59(4), 484–506.

1. Baker, *The Medical Malpractice Myth*; Gibson and Singh, *Wall of Silence: The Untold Story of the Medical Mistakes That Kill and Injure Millions of Americans.*
2. Millenson, "The Silence"; Baker, *The Medical Malpractice Myth.*
3. Baker, *The Medical Malpractice Myth.*
4. Ibid.
5. Ibid.
6. *Defensive Medicine and Medical Malpractice*, 1.
7. Studdert D.M. et al., "Defensive Medicine among High-Risk Specialist Physicians in a Volatile Malpractice Environment."
8. Ibid.
9. Ibid.
10. Baker, *The Medical Malpractice Myth.*
11. Ibid.; Wachter and Shojania, *Internal Bleeding*; America et al., *To Err Is Human.*
12. *House of Cards.*
13. *Fear of Flying.*
14. *Under Control.*
15. *Shifts Happen.*
16. *Such Sweet Sorrow.*
17. *The Crossing.*
18. *The Visit.*
19. Shore, *The Mistake.*
20. *Fear of Flying.*
21. *The Self-Destruct Button.*
22. *The Ethics of Hope.*
23. Rimes, *Shake Your Groove Thing.*
24. *Post Mortem.*
25. Crichton, *Out of Africa.*
26. Horwitz, Green, and Bradley, "US Emergency Department Performance on Wait Time and Length of Visit."
27. Iezzoni et al., "Survey Shows That At Least Some Physicians Are Not Always Open Or Honest With Patients."
28. Ibid.
29. Millenson, "The Silence."

30. Ibid.

31. Baker, *The Medical Malpractice Myth.*

32. Martins, "Experiences of Homeless People in the Health Care Delivery System"; Hudson et al., "Health-Seeking Challenges Among Homeless Youth."

33. Martins, "Experiences of Homeless People in the Health Care Delivery System."

34. Kushel et al., "Emergency Department Use Among the Homeless and Marginally Housed"; Kushel, M.B., Vittinghoff, E., and Haas, J.S., "Factors Associated with the Health Care Utilization of Homeless Persons."

35. Hudson et al., "Health-Seeking Challenges Among Homeless Youth."

36. *Lamb to the Slaughter.*

37. *House Training.*

38. *When the Bough Breaks.*

39. Rimes, *Shake Your Groove Thing.*

40. Shore, *Daddy's Boy.*

41. *Humpty Dumpty.*

42. *Fidelity.*

43. *Three Stories.*

44. Baer, "Cardiopulmonary Resuscitation on Television. Exaggerations and Accusations"; "How Authentic Is Medicine on Television?".

45. America et al., *To Err Is Human.*

46. Blendon et al., "Views of Practicing Physicians and the Public on Medical Errors"; Wachter and Shojania, *Internal Bleeding.*

47. Gibson and Singh, *Wall of Silence: The Untold Story of the Medical Mistakes That Kill and Injure Millions of Americans.*

Chapter Five

"If you had only..."

"Preventable" Conditions and Patient Responsibility

As a society, we expect American consumers to take responsibility for their health: eat healthy foods, exercise, practice safe sex and follow other recommended behaviors, with the assumption that all consumers are capable of adapting these lifestyle changes and that these behaviors will protect a person from ill health. This focus on personal responsibility has hindered programs to help individual consumers improve their health and has reinforced stigma about those with "preventable" conditions. How do we learn what behaviors are healthy or how to play the role of patient? Health campaigns, advertising, and news media have certainly promoted personal responsibility. Even more so, though, entertainment television has perpetuated this approach to healthcare, modeling a doctor-patient relationship (albeit fictional) in which patients are held responsible for becoming ill or injured. This chapter explores the patient's role in fictional dramas, examining the extent to which characters are blamed for their "preventable" conditions.

The patients' role in medical dramas has been largely overlooked. Most studies on these programs have focused on the fictional physician or other aspects of the genre.[1] The overall absence of research in this area may be explained by the traditional "doctor show" formula, in which dramas have showcased the heroics of the doctor, while downplaying the role of the patient in medical care. Patients were responsible for little more than showing up to the doctor's office. In the 1970s, fictional television largely ignored preventative medicine. For example, although the link between smoking and cancer had been well-established, the medical drama *Marcus Welby, M.D.* frequently depicted characters smoking cigarettes. In one episode, Dr. Welby even lights the cigarette of a patient's wife in the hospital hallway, with no discussion of the possible risks. Contemporary medical dramas focus much more on the fictional patients. With this inclusion, the patients' behavior also becomes part of the storyline. This chapter looks at fictional patient cases of "preventable" medical conditions, as a means to examine the relationship between public discourse on personal responsibility and its media images.

PATIENTS HELD RESPONSIBLE FOR ILL HEALTH

We perceive certain health conditions as, at least, somewhat "preventable" in that particular behaviors heighten one's risk of developing the condition. In contemporary medical dramas, health professionals frequently blame patients for their "preventable" conditions after they had engaged in "risky" behaviors, including substance abuse, poor diets, unsafe sexual practices, violence, the failure to use seatbelts and other foolish actions.

Substance Abuse

Reflective of real-life, medical dramas convey that substance abuse led to an array of health problems. Smoking is the most common "risky" behavior, causing patients to develop lung cancer, emphysema, heart disease, and other health problems. The risk of smoking to oneself and others has been recognized in federal and state legislation, first in its television advertising ban, and in recent restrictions on smoking in public restaurants and other places. [2] Although it is common knowledge that smoking increases risks, approximately 46 million people (20.6 percent of the population) smoke. [3] According to the Centers for Disease Control, smoking is the number one cause of preventable death. [4]

Medical drama storylines primarily showcase the danger of smoking for the individual (as opposed to second or third hand smoke). In a serial storyline, beginning in season four in *ER*, smoking slowly destroys the life of Dr. Mark Greene's father, David. During the introduction of this character, Dr. Greene catches his father smoking in the garage and lectures him on the dangers, especially because his father already has a chronic cough and emphysema. A few seasons later, David is diagnosed with lung cancer, which transforms him from an active, healthy person to a thin, frail figure in a hospital bed, who soon passes away. By showing Greene's father smoking, his diagnosis of lung cancer, and his final days, this storyline illustrates the long-term effects of tobacco use on one's health and depicts Greene's father as responsible for his early death.

Another episode of *ER* about smoking is somewhat comical when a heavy smoker suggests that he is not responsible for his medical condition. In "No Good Deed Goes Unpunished," [5] Dr. Luka Kovac diagnoses a patient, Mr. Carmichael, with a form of lung cancer.

Mr. Carmichael: I need you to write me up a full disclosure so I can file a
lawsuit against the tobacco companies.
Kovac: Mr. Carmichael, you've been smoking cigarettes since you were a
teenager.
Carmichael: So?

Mr. Carmichael uses a nebulizer to help him breathe as Kovac stares at him.

Kovac: So you have to take some responsibility for that. Instead of looking for
someone else to blame, you should be concentrating on how to manage your
disease and make the most out of the time you have left.

Mr. Carmichael coughs and gasps for air.

Mr. Carmichael: I get it. It's just the HMOs and big business covering each
other's asses. Well, screw you pal. I'll see you in court.
Kovac: No, you won't.
Mr. Carmichael: Oh yeah? You don't think I won't sue you, too?
Kovac: You're not going to live that long.

The dialogue and Kovac's reaction to the patient's attempt to blame others
for his medical condition construct the patient as truly responsible—and as
someone who should take responsibility for his illness.

Smoking also causes other health problems for fictional patients. In the
Grey's Anatomy episode "Tell Me Sweet Little Lies,"[6] surgeons tell a teenage guitar player that his newly reattached fingers will likely turn necrotic
due to poor circulation if he does not quit smoking. And, in another episode,
a patient on oxygen lights a cigarette, causing an explosion, badly burning
him. The Chief of Surgery, Dr. Webber, comments, "What kind of idiot
lights a cigarette in a hospital?" In these storylines, the fictional health professionals lecture patients on the dangers of smoking, without providing
much information on how to quit. Futhermore, the depiction of the smoking
teenager was a missed opportunity to address the problem of adolescent
cigarette use. Since more than 80 percent adult smokers started before age
eighteen, exploring the external factors that influence teenage initiation
might help deter youth smokers.[7]

Fictional patients are also held responsible for illness and injuries caused
by alcohol abuse. Prosocial media messages about the dangers of alcohol can
be traced back to the Harvard Alcohol Project of the mid-1980s, which first
introduced (quite successfully) the concept of the "Designated Driver."[8]
Contemporary programs highlight the possible risks of alcohol abuse. Short-
term consequences typically were portrayed with college drinking and included alcohol poisoning and injuries, followed by reprimands from the
treating health professionals. In the *ER* episode, "Into That Good Night,"[9] a
Caucasian male college student almost dies after he participates in a binge-

drinking game. When the student wakes up after treatment, Dr. Susan Lewis lectures him on his dangerous behavior, saying, "You're on dialysis because you drank too much. Blink if you will never do this again." The student blinks, indicating that he understands that his behavior was risky. And in "Dr. Carter, I Presume,"[10] a drunken man needs hundreds of stitches after he falls through a plate glass window. Medical students joke about how long it will take to stitch the man up, augmenting both the foolishness and consequences of the man's actions.

Chronic alcohol abuse storylines use much more somber tones, with depictions of the effects of liver disease and other problems. The *ER* episode "Time of Death"[11] focused exclusively on the last hour of a patient's life as he slowly dies from liver failure. It begins with a patient, Charlie Medcaff (played by Ray Liotta, who won an Emmy for this role), collapsing in the emergency room waiting room. The doctors determine that he is bleeding internally and will soon die. Dr. Greg Pratt questions helping the patient, saying, "We're killing ourselves for a noncompliant, alcoholic, end-stage liver failure drifter." Later in the episode, Pratt and the other doctor, Dr. Kovac, argue about the man's responsibility for his condition.

> Pratt: The guy's a waste. He's dying from something he did to himself.
> Kovac: Last time I checked, alcoholism is a disease.
> Pratt: So's suicide. He should catch some of that and save us the trouble.
> Kovac: We get one like this everyday.

Flashbacks showcase consequences of the man's drinking, including his prison time for killing a man in a bar fight and losing custody of his child. The doctors call Charlie's son, who tells Charlie, "Nice knowing you" and hangs up on him. Following this rejection, Charlie begins to sob as he recalls the events in his life.

The physical effects of the alcohol on Charlie are shown throughout the episode. Charlie is pale, with bloodshot, watery eyes. Shortly after admission, Charlie is shown with blood draining out of his mouth through a tube. Later, as doctors place a scope down Charlie's throat, his damaged bleeding intestines appear on a screen. The doctors inform Charlie that he needs a new liver, which he will not receive because of his history of drinking. At this point, Charlie asks them to stop treatment. To keep him comfortable, doctors give Charlie an IV of alcohol. In the final moments of the episode, Charlie goes into cardiac arrest and dies alone. Charlie's life flashbacks and final hour painfully demonstrate the devastating health and social consequences of alcohol abuse. An estimated 79,000 people die each year from excessive alcohol.[12] And yet, while the dangers alcoholism are shown, the reasons why people binge drink or abuse alcohol in other ways (i.e., because of peer pressure or depression) are not addressed, nor are the resources available for those who want to stop, like Alcoholics Anonymous. The link between alcohol abuse and liver failure has been shown to influence the extent to which doctors believe that alcoholics deserve liver transplants. [13]

Narcotic use is portrayed as having more permanent consequences for patients. In season four of *ER*, Dr. John Carter learns that his cousin, Chase, is addicted to heroin. In "Sharp Relief," [14] Carter helps Chase through withdrawal as he attempts to overcome his heroin addiction. Four episodes later, Chase relapses and is brought to the hospital after injecting tainted heroin. Chase stops breathing and is deprived of oxygen, causing severe brain damage. Several seasons later, Carter becomes addicted to narcotics from medication he received after being brutally stabbed in the hospital. When his friends encourage him to seek help, he resists. Dr. Benton says to Carter, "What is it in you man, huh? This week Fentanyl, next week you end up dead or worse, like your cousin, as some babbling gork in a nursing home?" With the thought of Carter's addiction causing him to become like Chase, Carter starts crying and agrees to enter rehabilitation for his addiction to narcotics.

In addition to showing the negative health effects for the drug users, the *ER* episode "Under Control" [15] conveyed the tragic consequences of a mother's amphetamine use on her infant. In this episode, the medical team struggles to revive an infant in cardiac arrest but cannot save her. After the baby dies, Dr. Greene learns that amphetamines in the baby's system caused seizures and cardiac arrest. Greene and Nurse Hathaway ask the baby's mother about the drugs.

> Mother: I work two jobs. Sometimes I get so tired, I take something to stay awake but I never bring drugs home.
> Hathaway: Are you nursing the baby?
> The woman nods.
> Greene: The drugs are in the breast milk.
> Mother (cries): I love my baby. I would never hurt her. I didn't know. Really, I didn't know.

Although this scene conveys the difficulty of being a poor working mother, the connection between her drug use and the baby's death from cardiac arrest constructs the mother as responsible for her behavior and its tragic consequences. While these stories are certainly heart-wrenching, these cautionary scenes offer little hope for viewers already addicted to substances. Other than Carter's narcotics rehabilitation experience (at a place for physicians only), these dramas lack information on how to avoid addiction, as well as resources on ending addictive behaviors.

Obesity

One-third of adult Americans are considered obese. [16] Even more alarming, is that the number of overweight adolescents has tripled in the last thirty years. [17] Meredith Minkler explained that this obesity crisis in America demonstrates the ineffectiveness of personal responsibility messages. [18] The connection between obesity (or diet) and ill health was often portrayed in contemporary medical dramas, in which the dialogue linked obesity to coronary disease, diabetes and hypertension.

In "Faith," [19] a sixty-four-year-old Caucasian woman complains of abdominal pain to Dr. Carter, who attributes her discomfort to her diet. The woman tells Carter that she had her "usual" breakfast—"Three fried eggs, bacon, glass of buttermilk, toast with jam." He replies, "Ah, the American Heart Association breakfast." The woman quickly retorts, "Don't lecture me doctor. My mother had the exact same breakfast every day of her life. Died last year at ninety-six. Car accident." The woman is brought to surgery for her abdominal pain and her prognosis is unknown. Carter's reaction, however, implicates the woman in her poor health.

In *ER*, the emergency room desk clerk, Frank, is overweight and often eats unhealthy foods at work. In season ten, Frank experiences a heart attack in the episode "Forgive and Forget." [20] When Dr. Pratt hears that Frank needs help, he says, "What did he do now? Choke on a donut?" As Pratt and other doctors struggle to lift Frank onto a gurney, Pratt complains, "He sucks down fried chicken for thirty years. Now we gotta pay." Frank eventually recovers and returns to work. Frank's reputation for eating unhealthy foods, combined with Pratt's comments, connected his poor diet to his heart attack, constructing Frank as responsible for his ill health.

A patient's obesity as a risk factor is also emphasized in the *ER* episode "Get Carter," [21] in which a paramedic jokes about the patient's weight, telling the doctors that they might need steroids to lift him. A few scenes later, the man is plopped (accompanied by a loud "thud") on a bed in the trauma room. An overhead shot of the patient showcases his girth filling the width of the bed. The man begs, "Please, let me sit up. I can't catch my breath." Dr. Carter replies, "That's 'cause you've got too much weight on your chest." No further information is offered, suggesting that his weight alone is impairing his breathing.

In some cases, a patient's obesity distracts the health professionals from the correct diagnosis. The fictional doctors of *Chicago Hope* attribute a man's ill health to his obesity until tests indicate that he is actually malnourished. Two episodes of *House, M.D.*, convey a similar message as obesity obscures the actual diagnoses. After a young, overweight girl has a heart attack in the episode "Heavy," [22] Dr. Robert Chase remarks to another doctor, "If I was that fat, I'd be pretty tempted to knock back a bottle of pills." The girl's mother begs the doctors, "Why can't any of you doctors see past her weight? If diet and exercise are the treatment, then the diagnosis is wrong." House's team checks her for diabetes and blood clots (conditions associated with obesity). Finally, when the diagnostics team looks beyond her weight, they discover that she has Cushing's Syndrome, caused by a tumor on her pituitary gland. They remove the tumor, curing her symptoms, and she quickly slims down.

Likewise, the episode "Que Será, Será"[23] centers around extreme size of a morbidly obese man through the dialogue, visuals of the patient himself and the limitations on diagnosing him because of his weight. The episode begins with firefighters cutting a large hole in the wall of a house. The camera shot cuts to inside the house, where paramedics are shown attempting to lift a morbidly obese man.

> Fireman 1: What? Are you kidding me? Tub of goo there's got to be over six bills. You ain't gonna lift him with a couple of blankets.
> Fireman 2: Got a better idea, Einstein?
> Fireman 1: Yeah, just roll him off. [The others laugh]. What? He's already dead. Ain't like he's gonna feel it.
> Fireman 3: How the hell does a guy get that big?
> Paramedic: If you roll him off from this side, he's likely to go right through the floor and take us with him.

At the hospital, the dean of medicine, Dr. Lisa Cuddy, tells Dr. Alison Cameron about the patient, stating, "forty-six-year-old guy in a coma; doesn't appear to be anything wrong with him except for the fact that he weighs over 600 pounds." Cuddy adds that the patient's exact weight is unknown because "The biggest scale we've got only goes up to 350 but this guy's waistline is over 7 feet."

Despite the patient's weight, his diagnostic tests appear normal. Yet, in conversations with the other doctors, House calls the patient "a hippopotamus" and "Shamu." Dr. Chase says, "I doubt a guy who weighs 600 pounds bothers with annual physicals." The patient's weight is also emphasized in the obstacles that the diagnostics team faces in examining him. The team cannot give the patient a CT scan or an MRI because he is over the weight limit. Dr. Eric Foreman has difficulty wrapping the blood pressure cuff around the man's large arm. As Foreman struggles with the cuff, the discussion turns to the patient's choices.

> Foreman: It's hard to believe you can even attach this much flesh to a human skeleton.
> Chase: I wouldn't exactly call this attached. This is ridiculous. A person shouldn't be able to eat themselves into oblivion and then just expect everyone to pull out the stops to fix everything.

> Foreman: What are we supposed to do? Refuse treatment to anyone who's obese?
> Chase: Come on, give me a break. This guy isn't obese. He's not even morbidly obese. He's suicidal.
> Foreman: Well, people who attempt suicide get treated.
> Chase: But yet non-compliant diabetics don't. We don't give drug addicts dialysis or alcoholics liver transplants.

By the end of the episode, House and the diagnostics team determine that the patient has lung cancer that has matastisized to his brain—unrelated to his weight. However, the abundant comments and limitations of diagnosing such a heavy patient indicate that had he been slimmer, the cancer may have been diagnosed sooner.

Diet appears to be a double-edged sword in medical dramas. When people ate poorly, they became obese and suffered ill health. At the same time, the dramas connected patients' efforts at weight loss to serious medical conditions, including cardiac problems, infections and vitamin deficiencies. In the *Chicago Hope* episode "Broken Hearts,"[24] a pregnant woman needs a heart transplant after her diet pills damaged her heart. In "Leggo My Ego,"[25] a male teenage wrestler becomes anorexic, which damages his heart, requiring surgery. Doctors then lecture him of the dangers of his eating disorder.

Weight-loss surgery also causes damaging health effects for fictional patients. In the *Grey's Anatomy* episode "The Self-Destruct Button,"[26] a mother pressures her college-aged daughter to maintain her slim physique. As a desperate solution, the young woman travels to Mexico for gastric bypass surgery, leading to a devastating infection. The surgeons at Seattle Grace remove a large portion of her bowel and speculate that she will never lead a normal life again. Likewise, a young woman's desire to be thin leads to paralysis and other neurological problems in the *House, M.D.* episode "Meaning."[27] Dr. Eric Foreman informs the woman, Caren, that she has scurvy and describes its effects:

> Foreman: Your arm and leg tissues are choked with blood. Makes it hard to move. Also damages your hair and toenails.
> Caren: But I'm on this great diet, lots of protein, lots of—
> Foreman: No vitamin C.

Foreman hands Caren a glass of orange juice and orders, "Now drink." The vitamin C in the juice cures her scurvy and she recovers from her paralysis.

These episodes construct people as responsible for their medical conditions if they follow poor diets or choose foolish means to lose weight. Most people know that eating unhealthy foods can lead to an array of medical problems. Yet, as Chip and Dan Heath pointed out in the best-selling book *Switch: How to Change Things When Change is Hard*, the U.S. govern-

ment's food pyramid and similar campaigns have failed to dramatically reduce obesity because they do not offer tangible alternatives.[28] Thus, as Heath
and Heath discussed, offering practical solutions, like the "1 percent or less"
campaign (encouraging people to buy 1% milk) could prompt viewers to
make a healthy change.[29]

The Consequences of Unsafe Sex

Even with widespread awareness of the risks of unprotected sex, an estimated 19 million infections are newly diagnosed each year, nearly half among
those were age fifteen to twenty-four.[30] While storylines about sex did not
often appear in older medical dramas, "unsafe" sex messages were conveyed
in dramas of the 1990s and beyond. Especially in *ER* (likely because it is set
at an urban, county hospital), sexual promiscuity often leads to unwanted
pregnancy and sexually transmitted diseases. Numerous fictional patients
were diagnosed with syphilis, HIV, HPV, and gonorrhea, manifested in the
throat, knee, heart, and other parts of the body. While most were successfully
treated, some patients faced long-term or fatal consequences for their actions.

In *ER*, some of the patients diagnosed with sexually transmitted disease
admitted to prostituting themselves, as exemplified in "Ground Zero."[31] Dr.
Anna Del Amico examines a patient named Vinnie, who has long black hair
and is wearing a brightly colored polyester shirt. After Del Amico diagnoses
Vinnie with gonorrhea, he tells her that the disease is an "Occupational
hazard. Price of being a playa." The patient expresses awareness of the
consequences but dismisses them as an acceptable risk.

Most of the fictional patients diagnosed with STIs were teenagers—a
trend which is reflective of real-life. The doctors instructed these patients on
how to protect themselves in the future. For example, Dr. Kovac diagnoses a
thirteen-year-old boy with chlamydia in the *ER* episode "Forgive and Forget,"[32] informing him about the disease and providing condoms. In another
storyline, a teenage girl develops cervical cancer as a result of contracting the
Human Papilloma Virus (HPV). This episode was part of a Kaiser Family
Foundation study, designed to educate viewers on the dangers of unsafe
sexual contact—and was proven effective.[33] A follow-up survey of viewers
found that 32 percent first learned about HPV from this storyline.[34] Even the
health care providers contracted STIs, despite their medical knowledge. Physician Assistant Jeanie Boulet contracts HIV from her cheating husband.
And, similar to a storyline in the pilot of *St. Elsewhere*,[35] in the *Grey's
Anatomy* episode "Who's Zoomin' Who?"[36] Drs. George O'Malley and Alex
Karev contract syphilis from a nurse. This spread of the sexually transmitted
disease conveys that even the health professionals do not practice safe sex.

A few cases exemplifiy the devastating effects of sexual promiscuity. In
the *ER* episode "You Bet Your Life,"[37] a Caucasian woman attempts suicide

because she contracted AIDS and passed it to her daughter, who then died of the disease. She is admitted after swallowing antifreeze, which has severely damaged her vision and will soon cause her death. The woman's ex-husband, Roger, discusses her condition with Jeanie Boulet.

> Roger: Is she in pain?
> Boulet: Some.
> Roger: Good. She cheated on me. Got herself infected with AIDS and gave it to our baby. I've been waiting for this for a long time.

In the woman's final moments, she becomes delirious and begs, "Please, Roger. Please, forgive me" even though Roger is not in the room. Later, the woman is shown dead. The patient's tragic final moments emphasize the magnitude of her irresponsible behavior. She has charcoal marks on her face and the disconnected intubation tube hangs from her mouth. Her eyes are vacant. Boulet cleans up her body, which is especially moving, given Jeanie's own HIV diagnosis.

The social consequences of having a sexually transmitted disease were conveyed in a few cases. In the episode "Food Chains" of *Chicago Hope*,"[38] emergency room doctor Danny Nylund passes over a critically injured woman after he learns that she has AIDS and instead attends to a patient with less serious wounds. Although Nyland is reprimanded, this case implied that fictional doctors, at least, may believe that some types of patients are more important to save than others. *ER* episodes also convey the social stigmas of certain "preventable" conditions. For example, Dr. Kerry Weaver covers up a respected alderman's diagnosis of syphilis (contracted from his male assistant). She treats the alderman without documenting the case and provides penicillin for his partner, whom she never examines. The case turns tragic when the partner has an allergic reaction to the penicillin and dies. Yet no one discovers Weaver's actions. And, as a reward for Weaver's discretion, the alderman donates millions of dollars to the hospital.

Many patients are constructed as sexually irresponsible. Because of their actions, these patients contracted sexually transmitted diseases and were lectured on their behavior. Yet, unlike some of the other "preventable" conditions, more information, including prevention, was included in storylines about STIs, likely because teenagers were often the focus. The HPV and other pro-social campaigns promoting teen sexual responsibility likely also influenced these messages.

Injuries from Violence

Some patients are constructed as responsible for injuries they incurred because their behavior put them at risk for harm. Participating in gang activity or criminal acts was connected to patients' injuries, for example. Storylines also suggest that careless behavior could put a patient at risk for victimization. In other words, the medical drama message is that patients would not have been injured if they had not put themselves at risk. Stories fictionalizing violent crime primarily appear in *ER* and *Chicago Hope*, which is not surprising, given their urban setting (downtown Chicago) and for *ER*, lower income clientele, in comparison to the posh hospitals of *House, M.D.* and *Grey's Anatomy*.

In *Chicago Hope* and *ER*, numerous patients had gunshot wounds they received while committing crimes or participating in gang activities. For example, in the *ER* episode "Feb. 5 '95,"[39] paramedics wheel in an African American boy who is covered with blood. A paramedic named Doris says, "Twelve year old male, multiple gunshot wounds to the leg and abdomen." As the doctors began to assess the boy's condition, Dr. Carter asks Doris about the boy's injuries.

> Carter: Drive-by?
> Doris: Drug deal gone bad. Gang bang.
> Carter: At 12 years old?
> Doris: Kid had a Tec-9 and a Luger on him when we found him.

Later in the episode, another African American boy walks through the emergency room, waving a gun. The boy enters the trauma room, where a heart-rate monitor is emitting a long sound, indicating that the first boy's heart has stopped. Dr. Benton tells the boy with the gun, "You're too late. He's already dead." The boy points the gun at Benton. He does not shoot, but runs out the room. Health professionals often comment on gang member patients as "frequent flyers" because of their repeated visits. In a few episodes, the patient is treated, left the hospital and then was brought back by paramedics with more serious wounds. In "Vanishing Act,"[40] Nurse Hathaway tries to convince a young African American man not to seek revenge for his superficial stab wounds. Against Hathaway's advice, the patient leaves the hospital. Hours later, paramedics bring the man in with multiple gunshot wounds and a collapsed lung. This patient's case, and others, suggested that participation in gang activity would eventually lead to severe injury or death.

The fictional doctors (sometimes falsely) associated violently injured African American male teenagers with gang activity. This assumption leads to delayed treatment of an African American gunshot victim in the *ER* episode "Tribes."[41] When two teenage gunshot victims are brought into the hospital, doctors assume that the African American patient was shot because of gang affiliations, while the Caucasian teenager was, as Dr. Greene says, "in the wrong place at the wrong time." They attend to the Caucasian teenager first, before the black patient, who dies in surgery. Later, the treating professionals learn that the African American teenager is an all-star high school basketball player. The Caucasian patient's parents tell the doctors that their son is a crack addict. This episode suggested that because of the doctors' perceptions of the patients, the Caucasian teenager received preferential treatment over the African American teenager.

Some medical drama storylines imply that some fictional female patients are constructed as responsible for their injuries if they place themselves in "dangerous" situations. Women are portrayed as at least partially responsible for their sexual assault if they had been "careless," such as with the security of their homes. Although the treating health professionals assured these patients that they are inculpable, the dialogue detailing their actions suggests otherwise. For example, in "Tribes,"[42] a college student believes that she had been raped, as the woman tells Nurse Hathaway, "I had a few beers at this party last night. I saw this guy, Mike, and I was going to give him a ride home. And then I woke up in my car in the dorm parking lot, my tights were off all the way and I don't know what happened." Hathaway finds out that the patient tested positive for the date rape drug. Upon being informed, the girl says, "Oh my God. How could I have been so stupid?" Hathaway responds, "You weren't stupid. Just trusted someone you shouldn't have." Yet, even though Hathaway finds evidence of rape and gives the patient antibiotics and emergency contraception, no police charges are discussed.

In "Think Warm Thoughts,"[43] a man rapes elderly women, mostly in their homes, and carves the word "whore" into their backs. In addition to the visual atrocity of this word upon the naked bodies of the elderly women, the horror of this experience is further emphasized by one victim's recollection of the attack. When she wakes up in the emergency room, the woman, Mrs. Reilly, tells Nurse Hathaway of her assault.

> Mrs. Reilly: I left my keys in the door and a man walked into my apartment.
> Hathaway: Mrs. Reilly?
> Mrs. Reilly: And he put his hand up over my mouth and he made me get down
> on the ground.

The patient begins to cry. Nurse Hathaway holds Mrs. Reilly and comforts her. Other elderly women also fall victim to the rapist, and in the subsequent episode "Sharp Relief,"[44] an elderly woman is found unconscious with the word "whore" carved into her back. This victim, who was brutally stabbed, dies of her wounds. The dire consequences for this woman and other victims emphasize the gravity of failing to take precautions. By offering the information that the intruder entered through an unlocked door, the storylines convey these victims as bearing some responsibility for their attacks.

The attribution of blame to victims of crime can have serious implications. To stereotype African American teenagers as "gang-bangers," for example, may mean that patients that fit this type may be perceived as "thugs" even if they are not part of this group. And, of course, assigning blame to female victims of sexual assault perpetuates a common rape myth—that this type of victim somehow "asks" to be raped. The extent to which people believe that a victim somehow contributed to the crime can affect public support for the victim, restitution, and the judicial process, as well as influencing stereotypes and the power dynamics of a society.[45] In medicine, this victim blame may translate to patient care, especially if some patients are more valued over others.

Failure to Use Protective Equipment

Patients are shown as responsible for their medical conditions when they experience serious injuries because they do not take the proper precautions. For some patients, it is implied that their injuries would have only been minor had they worn their seatbelts. In the *Grey's Anatomy* episode "Enough is Enough (No More Tears),"[46] a surgeon states, "I don't know why people think they don't need seatbelts," as he operates on a severely injured automobile accident victim. Doctors lecture a patient with internal bleeding on the use of seatbelts in *ER* episode "Feb. 5 '95."[47] Dr. Peter Benton asks the man, "Were you wearing your seatbelt?" When he replies, "No," Nurse Hele says, "You will the next time, I bet." Hele's comment emphasizes this link, conveying that the patient should learn from his mistakes and protect himself in the future. These messages are consistent with campaigns like "Click It or Ticket" that promote safe equipment. The risks of cell phone use were not addressed in the fictional messages, despite the 28 percent increase in deaths from distracted driving between 2005 and 2008.[48] Such issues would be especially relevant for contemporary programming.

Foolish Actions and "Preventable" Injuries

Much of the humor in medical dramas emerges when fictional patients sustain minor injuries participating in rather foolish activities. In "Family Matters"[49] of *ER*, a young woman breaks both ankles jumping into a polar bear pit for a scavenger hunt picture. In "Insurrection," two men sever fingers while attempting to trim a hedge with a lawnmower. The hospital staff misplaces the men's severed fingers. When they locate the bag, Dr. Chen complains that no one sorted the fingertips. The focus is on the fingertips, as neither the patients' reattachment surgeries, nor the recoveries are shown. Similarly, in the episode "Missing,"[50] another patient severed his fingers when he tried to cut through ice with a chainsaw. Out of earshot, Nurse Sam Taggart derisively calls him a "genius."

Sexual injuries also provide humor in the programs. In the *ER* episode, "The Providers,"[51] a doctor attributes a man's sore penis to excessive masturbation. Fictional patients also needed treatment for objects wedged in body orifices. In "Insurrection,"[52] a man needs treatment for the large vibrator lodged deep in his rectum. Other health professionals watch and laugh as a new medical student attempts to pull out the device. In "Occam's Razor,"[53] a patient sees Dr. House because he cannot get an MP3 player out of his rectum. House mocks the young man's actions, asking him, "Is it because of the size, or the shape, or the pounding bass line?"

In "Oh the Guilt" of *Grey's Anatomy*, [54] two people get caught having an extra-marital affair when they become intertwined during intercourse and cannot free themselves. The treating physicians determine that the man's penile piercing caught on the woman's IUD and that the connected parts became lodged in her uterus. As the doctors untangle the couple, the man has a heart attack and needs immediate surgery. In the course of the episode, the man faces embarrassment and then has to undergo surgery for his indiscretions.

Because the storylines about sex are used for humor, they may discourage people with seemingly embarrassing conditions to seek medical treatment, fearing ridicule. People may delay treatment or attempt to treat themselves (possibly making their conditions worse) if they believe that health professionals will criticize their behavior.

WHO ISN'T RESPONSIBLE FOR A "PREVENTABLE" CONDITION?

As in real-life, not every fictional patient could have prevented his/her medical condition. Medical conditions that are depicted as being "non-preventable" include some cases of heart disease, diabetes, cancers other than lung cancer (i.e., pancreatic cancer), and genetic diseases like cystic fibrosis. In many cases, patients' injuries are portrayed as "non-preventable." For example, in one episode of *ER*, a woman is shown inspecting her bumper after she was rear-ended. As she is standing on the side of the road, between her car and the one that hit her, the car behind the woman is rear ended, pinning the woman between the two cars and severing her legs.

In some cases, particularly in the drama *Chicago Hope*, fictional patients are not depicted as responsible for their medical conditions because no information about patients' histories were connected to their medical conditions. Similar to *Marcus Welby, M.D.* and older dramas, by providing no information about the patient's history and showing no fictional professionals lecture patients about their past or future behavior, this medical drama suggests that most patients could not have prevented their disease or injury by abstaining from substances, eating better, practicing safe sex or engaging in other healthy behaviors. Even patients with sexually transmitted diseases are not typically lectured about safe sex. For example, a HIV-positive woman asks

Dr. Diane Grad for medical advice regarding pregnancy. Throughout her pregnancy and delivery, the woman's HIV status is discussed, but how she contracted the disease is never mentioned.

Few storylines highlight institutional flaws that lead to "preventable" medical conditions. Storylines depicted some patients as not responsible because their social circumstances are portrayed as hindering their ability to make responsible health choices. In *ER's* "Into That Good Night,"[55] pediatrician Dr. Doug Ross criticizes a poor African American woman for not giving her daughter her asthma medication. The daughter is having difficulty breathing. He tells the mother, "She could have died, don't you understand?" The mother explains that she could not afford the medication until her next paycheck. Ross goes to the pharmacy, purchases the medication, and personally delivers it to the woman and her daughter in their poor neighborhood, demonstrating that Ross realizes that it is the woman's economic status, not poor lifestyle decisions, that hinders her ability to help her daughter. This storyline hints at problems with a health care system that does not provide available care and medication.

In season six of *ER*, the episode "Loose Ends"[56] constructs an older African American diabetic man with a gangrenous leg as not responsible for his condition, even though the storyline conveyed that his diabetes had been poorly managed. Dr. Peter Benton tells the patient that his leg will probably have to be amputated. Instead of lecturing the patient, though, Benton holds another emergency room doctor responsible for the patient's condition. Dr. Luca Kovac had treated the patient a month before and had given him medication and a referral for a specialist to help the patient manage his diabetes. Benton criticizes Kovac, arguing that Kovac should have called the patient at home to make sure that he received follow-up care. This conversation conveyed that Benton holds Kovac, not the patient, responsible:

> Benton: Older African American men are at high risk for amputation because they're not treated aggressively. You should know that.
> Kovac: I do.
> Benton: Well, then, why didn't you call him?
> Kovac: What are you saying?
> Benton: I'm saying that there's more to emergency medicine than treating and streeting patients.
> Kovac: That's one more thing you don't have to teach me.

This storyline constructs the patient as not responsible for his poorly managed diabetes. Rather, the storyline portrayed that Kovac should have known that the patient, as an older African American man, needed more follow-up because of his age and race. Although the blame here is placed on Kovac, this storyline subtly addresses the drawbacks of a decentralized system of care.

The latter seasons of *ER* include more discussion of the role of social responsibility in health care. Questions of access to health care, the doctor's role in educating patients, and insuring follow-up care are brought up in a few patients' cases. As part of this discussion, a few storylines portrayed patients as not responsible for "preventable" medical conditions because obstacles hinder their ability to take measures to protect their health. These patients are typically portrayed as poor people who had recently immigrated to America.

In the episode "Get Carter,"[57] doctors diagnose a family of Haitian immigrants with whooping cough. In most storylines with people who contract diseases for which vaccines are available, doctors lectured the patients for failing to protect themselves against "preventable" diseases. Yet, for this case, no discussion of vaccines occurs in this episode, as the storyline centers on bringing the family and infected neighbors in for treatment. Even when the grandmother of the family dies from the illness, no doctors mention that her death could have been prevented. This case and a few others imply that flaws in the health care system need to be addressed in order for all people to practice good health behaviors.

CONCLUSION: THE IMPLICATIONS OF THE "(IR)RESPONSIBLE" PATIENT

Individual responsibility was heavily emphasized in the storylines of contemporary medical dramas. The pervasiveness of this model in storylines of the medical dramas suggests one way the notion of individual responsibility for health has been perpetuated in one cultural site.[58] The fictional doctors and other health professionals repeatedly criticized patient behavior, suggesting that they would not need medical treatment had they not participated in risky behavior, waited to go to the hospital, listened to their doctors, or attempted to treat themselves.

Obviously, it is beneficial to the public for these programs to show the risk of certain behaviors on health. At the same time, for these storylines to convey the message that doctors will dismiss or even ridicule patients who partake in "risky" behaviors is problematic. Calling a patient an "idiot" on TV may discourage real-life smokers from seeking medical treatment. These storylines also individualize these problems, suggesting that vulnerable individuals become addicted or obese, or participate in unsafe sex, ignoring social contexts that also contribute to these behaviors. For example, with the obese fictional patients, the focus on diet.[59] ignores our commercial culture in which we are bombarded with messages advertising fast food. Much like the Kaiser Family Foundation HPV study, these episodes missed an opportunity to educate viewers about alternative healthy behaviors.[60]

As with the fictional health professionals, storylines in contemporary dramas highlight the mistakes of the individual, while ignoring a flawed health care system that breeds medical errors and makes it difficult for people to adapt healthy behavior. Even more so than with the fictional doctors, patients were blamed for their poor decisions. This trend may be reflective of the historical stronghold of the medical profession on the "doctor shows."[61] Because real-life physicians have been involved with production, these programs favorably portray the health profession, even with *ER* and its followers.[62] Perhaps, then, in an effort to reflect the modern skepticism of health care without criticizing the institution, the medical shows of the *ER* era redirect the focus to the individual, thus using the patient as a scapegoat.

The personal responsibility model makes fiscal sense and may be effective for well-educated, higher socio-economic people who can afford gym memberships, healthy food, and other luxuries that help with maintaining good health. However, this approach ignores some African American and other groups that have historically distrusted health professionals, as well as those who do not understand "risky" behavior, or lack of childcare, transportation, or health insurance, and other fallacies of the personal responsibility model. Some may argue that the function of entertainment television is to entertain, not to educate. However, since these programs connect risky behavior to consequences, they are already creating opportunities to disseminate prosocial messages. Extensive research demonstrates that so-called "edu-tainment" programming is quite effective in influencing health knowledge and behavior.[63] That said, rather than just attributing blame, these programs could more effectively address the intrinsic and external factors that lead people to start and continue behavior that heightens their risks of injury or illness.

NOTES

1. Defleur, "Occupational Roles as Portrayed on Television"; MacDonald, "Black Doctors on Television"; McLaughlin, "The Doctor Shows"; Gerbner et al., "Health and Medicine on Television"; Pfau, Mullen, and Garrow, "The Influence of Television Viewing on Public Perceptions of Physicians"; Chory-Assad and Tamborini, "Television Doctors"; Turow, *Playing Doctor*.

2. "Smoking Bans Cut Number of Heart Attacks, Strokes."

3. Health, "Smoking and Tobacco Use; Fact Sheet; Adult Cigarette Smoking in the United States;."

4. Ibid.

5. *No Good Deed Goes Unpunished.*

6. *Tell Me Sweet Little Lies.*

7. Health, "Smoking and Tobacco Use; Fact Sheet; Youth and Tobacco Use."

8. Winsten, "Promoting Designated Drivers."

9. *Into That Good Night.*

10. Crichton, *Dr. Carter, I Presume.*

11. Crichton, *Time of Death.*

12. "CDC - Fact Sheets-Alcohol Use And Health - Alcohol."

13. Glannon, "Responsibility, Alcoholism, and Liver Transplantation."

14. Crichton, *Sharp Relief.*

15. *Under Control.*

16. Ogden et al., "Prevalence of Obesity in the United States, 2009–2010."

17. "Obesity and Overweight for Professionals."

18. Minkler, "Personal Responsibility for Health?"

19. *Faith.*

20. Crichton, *Forgive and Forget.*

21. *Get Carter.*

22. *Heavy.*

23. Shore, *Que Será Será.*

24. Kelley, *Broken Hearts.*

25. *Leggo My Ego.*

26. Rimes, *The Self-Destruct Button.*

27. *Meaning.*

28. Heath, *Switch.*

29. Reger et al., "1% or Less."

30. "STD Trends in the United States, 2010."

31. *Ground Zero.*

32. Crichton, *Forgive and Forget.*

33. Brodie et al., "Communicating Health Information Through The Entertainment Media."

34. Ibid.

35. Dr. Ben Samuels informs several nurses that he has gonorrhea and that they should also get tested.

36. *Who's Zoomin' Who?.*

37. *You Bet Your Life.*

38. Food Chains" of *Chicago Hope.*

39. *Feb. 5, '95.*

40. *Vanishing Act.*

41. *Tribes.*

42. Ibid.

43. *Think Warm Thoughts.*

44. Crichton, *Sharp Relief.*

45. Karmen, *Crime Victims*; Brownmiller, *Against Our Will.*

46. *Enough Is Enough (No More Tears).*

47. *Feb. 5, '95.*

48. Wilson and Stimpson, "Trends in Fatalities From Distracted Driving in the United States, 1999 to 2008."

49. *Family Matters.*

50. *Missing.*

51. *The Providers.*

52. *Insurrection.*

53. *Occam's Razor.*

54. *Oh, the Guilt.*

55. *Into That Good Night.*

56. *Loose Ends.*

57. *Get Carter.*

58. Turow (2010) argued that even contemporary medical shows have been apolitical, ignoring context.

59. Minkler, "Personal Responsibility for Health?"

60. Brodie et al., "Communicating Health Information Through The Entertainment Media."

61. Turow, *Playing Doctor.*

62. Ibid.

63. Winsten, "Promoting Designated Drivers"; Brodie et al., "Communicating Health Information Through The Entertainment Media"; Glik et al., "Health Education Goes Hollywood."

Chapter Six

"But Dr., I read online that. . ."

Patient Responsibility for "Non-preventable" Conditions

The previous chapter explored patient responsibility for health conditions considered "preventable." Obviously, not all conditions are connected to behaviors, as disease can also be caused by the environment, genetics, germs, or unknown factors. And yet, even when the condition is not preventable, patients can still be held responsible for seeking medical care when they notice health problems and managing chronic conditions. Patients have been increasingly expected to take an active role in the health care process as research in preventative medicine has expanded to include more behaviors that could impact health, ultimately shifting attention to the individual consumer.[1] Thus, the dominant model for the doctor-patient relationship began to shift from a paternalistic model to a doctor-patient relationship that encouraged patient participation.[2] This chapter focuses on the extent to which contemporary medical dramas portray this "active patient," exploring cases in which the fictional patients diagnosed or treated themselves, challenged their health professionals, or asserted themselves in other ways in the process of medical treatment. Representations of the doctor-patient relationships are discussed, including the expectations for patients in seeking treatment, maintaining health and following doctors' orders.

BACKGROUND: THE CHANGING DOCTOR-PATIENT RELATIONSHIP

Along with shifting ideologies about medicine and authority, vast improvements in technology over the last two decades have encouraged patient participation in health care. As of 2007, more than 122 million American people have used the Internet to find information about a personal health issue—a number that is growing.[3] From a patient's perspective, this usage has been largely beneficial. Internet usage has helped many people to feel more informed about their health and better understand their medical conditions or illnesses.[4] Patients who use the Internet for health information have reported feeling more engaged in their health and more confident about conversing with their physicians.[5] Online information can clarify or supplement a diagnosis or treatment and provide support for a medical condition, which can be especially helpful with embarrassing or stigmatized ailments.[6]

Despite a growing belief that increasing patient participation improves health care, the medical profession has not fully adopted this approach.[7] With the recent trend of parents electing not to immunize, for example, a 2005 study found that 39 percent of pediatricians surveyed would discontinue care with families who refused vaccinations, even with the argument that continued care with open communication about vaccinations would be a more beneficial approach.[8] This finding is not surprising, given that some physicians fail to discuss any concerns. M. Kim Marvel and colleagues observed physician-patient interactions, finding that physicians quickly redirected conversation when patients voiced concerns, without fully responding to their issues.[9] As a whole, physicians appear to be conflicted on the value of the "informed" patient model. Some physicians surveyed positively perceived those who learned about their health conditions online, provided they did not challenge the providers' authority.[10] On the other hand, physicians have questioned the credibility of online material, its potential for confusion, distress or harm for the patient, and time spent on irrelevant questions because of Internet usage.[11] Doctors have also expressed concerns that their authority is challenged and therefore may be reluctant to discuss online information and share in the decision-making process—a fear that is not unfounded.[12] A 2007 study by Envision Solutions found that 62 percent of people surveyed have doubted a physician's diagnosis or medical opinion that contradicted online information.[13] And yet, patients usually bring up online information to get the doctor's opinion, not to self-diagnose or to question the physician's authority.[14]

THE PATIENT ROLE IN CONTEMPORARY DRAMAS

Despite the increasing importance of the "active patient" in real-life, contemporary medical dramas present a far more negative view of this shifting relationship. Television's health professionals expect patients to live healthy lifestyles and to follow their advice. They lecture patients who lied or omitted important details of their medical history or seek medical treatment when they believe that it is not needed. For example, in *ER* and *House, M.D.*, health professionals advise patients in the waiting room to "go home" if they only have symptoms of the common cold or flu. And yet, the doctor-patient relationship modeled in these programs is paternalistic, negatively portraying patients who diagnosed themselves, administered treatment, or questioned their doctors.

As described in earlier chapters, medical dramas depict doctors as heroes who work on their patients' behalves. When the health professionals could continue their roles as advocates, the storylines positively portray active patients. For example, in "Wake Up"[15] and "Man with No Name"[16] of *ER*, a woman needs treatment for lead poisoning after she traveled to Mexico for preventative therapy against cancer. When this treatment makes her ill, her doctor, Abby Lockhart, brings up a preventative mastectomy. During surgery, doctors find enlarged lymph nodes in the woman, suggestive of cancer. Their discovery indicates that the woman was correct in seeking her own treatment. Similarly, in "Let it Be"[17] of *Grey's Anatomy*, a friend of Dr. Addison Montgomery begs her for a hysterectomy and mastectomy so that she will not succumb to cancer like many of her female relatives. Montgomery advises her friend on her decision, providing her with statistics about her risks. In these cases, the female doctors clearly empathize with the patients and counsel them on their decisions. Other active patients are portrayed positively when they are shown actively managing a chronic condition (or a family member's condition), provided they do not question the doctors or interfere with treatment.

NEGATIVE PORTRAYALS OF PATIENT ROLES IN HEALTH CARE

For the most part, patients dutifully followed their physicians' orders. However, when patients assert themselves, attempt to self-diagnose, or ask questions, they are criticized and face negative consequences for their actions. At the very least, most active patients annoyed their doctors. Multiple questions from a patient were conveyed as unnecessary and a poor use of the physician's time. For example, in *ER*'s "Let the Games Begin,"[18] a middle-age man asks Dr. Carter many questions. To irritate another doctor, Carter then recommends a local anesthetic for the man's operation so he can stay awake and ask questions during surgery. Carter's reaction suggests that asking questions is unusual and unnecessary. Likewise, Dr. House repeatedly mocks patients who question his diagnoses or treatments. In "TB or not TB,"[19] woman with cat allergies tells House that she does not want to take antihistamines or use nasal spray. House responds by telling her to kill the cat. In another episode, House ridicules a mother's amateur diagnosis of epilepsy for her daughter, informing her that the girl is actually masturbating. Because of House's reactions, patients seem hesitant to question his authority—especially because he almost always cures his patients. In real-life, many health professionals discourage the opinions and self-diagnosis of their patients. For example, Marvel and colleagues found that in clinical visits, physicians take over the conversation after approximately twenty-three seconds of greeting their patients, discouraging them from setting the agenda.[20] This study also found that some doctors do not solicit patients' concerns, instead simply make assumptions about the reasons for the visits.[21] This need for control runs counter to a patient participation model.

Patients' Behavior Delays Treatment

While patients are criticized for self-diagnosis, they are expected to be knowledgeable enough about disease to know when to seek treatment. Therefore, patients are constructed as responsible for ill health when they delay visiting their health care providers after noticing symptoms. The *ER* episode "Refusal of Care"[22] conveyed that a patient should have sought treatment sooner. Upon examination of an older African American woman, Dr. Greg Pratt finds a large tumor in her breast. She tells Pratt that she first noticed the lump a few years before. Dr. Ray Barnett asks the woman why she waited so long to see a doctor and tells her, "You could have caught this before it spread." Pratt adds, "Surgery may not be as effective at this advanced stage." She refuses to undergo surgery. Recognizing the woman's fear, Pratt brings in an advocate from a cancer support group who convinces the woman to have surgery. Showcasing this cancer support service may provide comfort to viewers who fear medical treatment, as research has shown that portraying this process can comfort viewers who share the condition.[23] At the same time, the criticism at the woman's initial examination may fuel existing fears. Even fictional doctors themselves fail to promptly seek care. In "Genevieve and the Fat Boy"[24] of *Chicago Hope*, Dr. Aaron Schutt diagnosis his colleague, Dr. Karen Antonovich with advanced skin cancer that has matastisized to her brain. Antonovich confesses that she first noticed symptoms months before, but had not sought medical treatment. Schutt informs her that the cancer is too advanced to be treated and she will soon die a painful death. In the next episode, Antonovich lapses into a coma and passes away.

When diagnosed with serious health conditions, real-life patients are encouraged and even expected to get a second opinion. Proponents of the Patient Advocate Foundation recommend seeking a second opinion for a medical diagnosis or course of treatment.[25] Yet, medical dramas portray this desire as foolish, even risky to the health of the patient. In the *ER* episode "Exodus,"[26] Dr. Ross diagnoses a young girl with renal failure due to *e. coli*, which he says she contracted from eating raw juice or sprouts. The mother initially refuses treatment, stating that she would like a second opinion. Ross tells her that she will die without immediate attention. When she finally consents, her daughter needs dialysis badly and nearly dies from renal failure in the hospital elevator. In another *ER* episode, "A Shot in the Dark,"[27] parents refuse to allow the surgeons to remove their daughter's appendix, insisting on her transfer to another hospital. When the girl's infection worsens, two doctors override the parents' consent, and remove the appendix just before it bursts. With the surgery a success, the parents calm down and explain their justification for the transfer. However, the surgeons' skill indicates that the transfer request was foolish and made the surgery much more risky. And in the *House* episode "Safe,"[28] parents forbid Dr. House from treating their teenage daughter because he had been wrong with previous attempts to diagnose her. Without consent, House examines the girl in the elevator, finding a tick in the girl's pubic hair. House faces no consequences for his actions and is praised by the girl's parents for curing their daughter. Even with exceptional care providers, research has noted significant discrepancies in both diagnoses and treatment plans, thus demonstrating the need for multiple opinions.[29] Recognizing its importance, most insurance plans, including Medicare, cover multiple opinions.[30]

Patients also delay treatment when doctors considered them too assertive. In five cases in the program *ER*, physicians dismissed persistent patients as hypochondriacs or drug-seekers. Sometimes called "frequent fliers," these patients did not always receive a medical examination or diagnostic tests. For example, in "Abby Road," after Nurse Abby Lockhart ignores a male patient's complaint of symptoms, the man has a heart attack. She justifies her mistake, stating that she believed he was a hypochondriac, and faces no consequences. In "Orion in the Sky,"[31] a man's personal physician missed a diagnosis of prostate cancer because he believed him to be fabricating his symptoms. By the time he visits the hospital, his cancer is very advanced, with a poor prognosis.

Health professionals also disregard patients who were perceived as too vocal about their pain. For example, in the *ER* episode "Rescue Me,"[32] Dr. Carter dismisses an African American man complaining about the severe pain in his leg, believing that he just wants narcotics. Thinking no one believes him, the man leaves. Carter then sees an ultrasound of the man's leg (taken by another doctor) and discovers a blood clot. He rushes out into the rain and finds the patient unconscious. Because of the delay, the clot traveled to his lung. The doctors perform a risky treatment and the man improves. Dr. House faced a similar experience, as described in the episode "Three Stories." His complaint about his pain delays his diagnosis by three days, causing the muscle tissue to die, leaving House with chronic pain. Real-world health professionals also struggle with identifying patients with drug-seeking behavior. One study found that complaining of intense pain is a strong predictor of narcotics abuse, suggesting that this portrayal is not unrealistic.[33] At the same time, this fictional dismissal may discourage real-life patients from describing severe pain, with the fear of being ignored or discriminated against.

Poor Management of Chronic Conditions

The Centers for Disease Control estimates that 50 percent of adults live with a chronic illness.[34] One in four adults has at least one limitation that affects daily life.[35] Furthermore, seven out of ten deaths in the United States are caused by chronic illnesses, many of which are preventable.[36] Despite this prevalence, fictional television negatively depicts those with chronic illness, holding them responsible for poor health when they did not properly manage their chronic medical conditions. For example, the *Grey's Anatomy* episode "Don't Stand So Close to Me"[37] conveys the devastating effects of poorly managed diabetes. An African American man in his thirties, Doug Kendry, complains of pain in his foot. Dr. Cristina Yang tells the man that, because he has diabetes, he should be inspecting his feet each day. Yang examines the patient and finds a large oozing sore on his foot. Yang determines that the infection has spread to the bone and that the foot needs to be amputated. She then suggests that the amputation could have been avoided if the patient had sought medical treatment sooner.

> Yang: Sir, diabetes is a manageable disease. If you had been here even a month ago, maybe...
> Doug: Okay, I screwed up. But you're telling me this is my only option because I was late getting in here? That there is no way...
> Yang: Mr. Kendry—
> Doug: No! Please, there's gotta be a way for me to get that month back. Tell me what to do. I'll do every line of every plan that you give me. Please. You gotta find a way to save my foot.

Later in the episode, Yang tells the other surgical interns about Doug's case, suggesting that he was responsible for the negative outcome.

> Yang: Hey, I have a type two diabetes. Patient let it go and the infection is in the bone. I have to find a fix or cut off the foot. Anyone? Anybody?
> Karev: You get to cut off his foot? Cool.
> Yang: Ok, no, not cool. The patient was neglectful. He made a couple bad calls. Does that mean he has no hope? Does that mean he can't have a do over?

Yang assists on the amputation of Doug's foot and she is shown cutting the femur. A little later, another doctor carries the severed diseased limb away from the patient. In the recovery room, Doug asks Dr. Yang what he should do now that he no longer has his leg. Yang responds, "You move forward. You follow the plan and you try and keep your other foot." This final comment to the patient indicates that Doug has some control over his future if he begins to carefully manage his diabetes, yet provides no information on how to safely manage diabetes to prevent further infection. According to the American Diabetes Association, an estimated 25.8 million people in the United States live with Diabetes.[38] Therefore, prosocial messages in these dramas could benefit many Americans. Patients were constructed as responsible for their ill health because they did not properly manage other conditions. In the *ER* episode "Great Expectations,"[39] an elderly African American woman becomes gravely ill after she skips her dialysis, because, she says, she wanted to get her hair done for her birthday. The excess fluid builds up around her heart and the woman dies. In *ER*'s "Last Call,"[40] a woman with epilepsy drinks tequila and uses cocaine. She goes into a coma and dies. Later, when the doctors inform the patient's sister of her death, the sister suggests that the patient was responsible for her actions, saying, "She knew she wasn't supposed to drink but that didn't stop her."

The programs *ER* and *Chicago Hope* each contain cases in which organ transplant recipients became severely ill because they did not properly manage their care. In the *ER* episode "Vanishing Act,"[41] Physician Assistant Jeanie Boulet determines that an older African American liver transplant recipient has severe liver damage. Boulet tells the man that because his drinking damaged his new liver, it is not likely that he will be eligible for another one. Similarly, the *Chicago Hope* episode "Second Chances"[42] focuses on a gravely ill middle-aged man who needs a new heart after he failed to take his daily regimen of medication for his first heart transplant. Because of the patient's poor management of his first transplant and his history of heroin abuse, he is not eligible for a second transplant and dies. This type of message may discourage viewers from becoming organ donors for fear that the recipients will fail to take care of the organs—one justification that people in real-life provide for refusing to become donors.[43] Considering that approximately 18 people on the transplant waiting list die each day, negative messages about organ donation have significant ramifications.[44]

The Danger of Self-treatment

People who tried to treat themselves were portrayed as foolish and often needed medical treatment for their choices. In *House*, a teenager develops neurological problems after taking anti-smoking remedies purchased online. Another patient mixes fertility drugs with birth control, causing a stroke and a liver tumor. In *ER*, a teenage boxer takes Ephedra, causing a brain bleed and death. Another boy injects growth hormones into his leg, resulting in an infection in his heart. Diet also causes health problems for patients. While patients are expected to eat healthy, extreme diets and dietary supplements cause patients' health distress, including heart failure from diet drugs, liver failure from poisonous mushrooms, scurvy due to an all-protein diet, and unplanned pregnancy because of the herb St. John's Wort.

Patients also attempt other "remedies" for perceived health conditions. In the *ER* episode "Insurrection,"[45] a woman attempts to manually remove her menstrual period, injuring her genitals. Dr. Luca Kovac explains the patient's case to Nurse Abby Lockhart.

> Kovac: Mrs. Lundgrum tried to vacuum out her period.
> Woman: Menstrual extraction is a very common practice.
> Lockhart: Practice for what?
> Woman: The day when the men who run the world take away your freedom of choice.
> Kovac: Til then, you could perforate your uterus, end up infertile, or bleed to death.
> Woman: If men needed abortions, there'd be drive-thrus with beer on tap and TVs tuned to ESPN.
> Lockhart: There's still no reason to do this to your body.
> Woman: You gotta wake up, honey. We're in a war.
> Lockhart: Conscientious objector.

This discussion implies that the patient's injury was a dangerous and risky practice, one that mocks feminists protests against patriarchy.

Other patients seek medical treatment after circumcising themselves with household tools, as in the *House, M.D.* episode "Autopsy."[46] House's reaction emphasizes the foolishness of the patient's actions.

> Patient: My new girlfriend had never been with a guy who wasn't c-circumcised so she freaked and—
> House: Aha, and you wanted Rivkah to feel all gemutlicht. I get it. It's a shandah.
> The patient drops his pants as House turns toward him.
> House: Gah!
> Patient: I got some box cutters and uh...
> House: Just like Abraham did it.
> Patient: I sterilized them, which, uh, I was told you're ...
> House: Stop talking. I'm gonna get a plastic surgeon. Get the Twinkie back in the wrapper.

House appears astounded at the man's actions as he leaves the room.

An episode of *ER* features a similar case, in which a young man circumcises himself and then comes to the hospital when he cannot stop the bleeding. In the emergency room, his girlfriend tells him that she had used her preference for circumcision only as an excuse to break up with him. Societal norms about circumcision have been changing in recent years. A 2013 study of circumcision trends noted a 10 percent decline over the last thirty years, demonstrating shifts in birth customs.[47]

Grey's Anatomy portrays two patients who disobey their doctors' orders and thus are responsible for the dire health consequences they face. In "Band Aid Covers the Bullet Hole,"[48] a patient named Heath, a hockey goalie, has a severe finger injury. Dr. Callie Torres bandages the finger and informs Heath that he needs surgery. Heath, who wants to delay surgery so that he can play in a hockey game that day, replies, "So here's what I'm thinking, we take this off; we put a small splint on my fingers so I can jam it into the glove. I play today and then I'm all yours!" Torres warns Heath of the potential danger of playing:

> Torres: Heath, if I cut that bandage off, we risk doing permanent damage to your finger. I'm with you, man, but I'm sorry. There's no way we can put your finger into a glove today.
> Heath: There must be something you can do. I need to play this afternoon. This game ... it's what I've been training for my entire life. This is my chance to go to college. This is my whole future.

Against Torres' advice, Heath leaves the hospital. Later in the episode, Heath enters the emergency room and walks up to Dr. O'Malley. Heath proudly tells O'Malley, "Hey. Told you I couldn't miss my game and I didn't. I made two goals and one assist and there were scouts there!" O'Malley notices that Heath has a blood-soaked towel wrapped around his hand. He asks him, "What did you do?" Heath replies, "I cut off my finger. It's okay. I saved it so you guys can sew it back on." Heath then shows O'Malley the severed finger packed in ice and tells him that he learned how to cut off his finger from a website.

The goalie's actions result in devastating consequences. As the surgeons reattach the finger, they discover a severe infection. Later, Drs. Torres and O'Malley inform Heath and his mother of his poor prognosis.

> Torres: When you put your freshly severed finger into a grungy-bacteria filled glove, you got a severe infection.
> Heath: What? No. The Internet didn't say anything about infection.
> O'Malley: Mrs. Mercer, we didn't realize how deep the infection had gone until we were in there. There was too much tissue damage.
> Torres: Heath, the infection was caused by a methicillin resistant staph bacteria and it's continuing to spread. We'll be lucky if we can preserve enough muscle for you to have any hand function at all.

Heath is shocked by the news and exclaims, "That's wrong. You're wrong. Ronnie Lott played for the 49ers when he cut off his finger. He could still play. I got the directions off the Internet. I..." Dr. Torres tells Health, "I'm sorry. I really am, but your hockey career is over." Heath's decision to go against medical advice costs him the function of his hand, sacrificing his hockey career, while highlighting the danger of treating oneself using online advice.

In "Tell Me Sweet Little Lies,"[49] a young Japanese competitive eater named Yumi has persistent hiccups. The doctors determine that she has a tear in the lining of her esophagus and needs surgery to repair it. Yumi's competitive eating coach, Mr. Kamaji, tells Dr. Bailey that Yumi is not available for surgery until after a competition that afternoon. Bailey replies, "No. Her schedule is clear now. She can't compete today. And if she enjoys the taste of solid food, I recommend giving up the sport for something a little less aggressive. Say boxing." Against medical advice, Yumi and her coach leave the hospital.

Later, intern Dr. Stevens informs Bailey that paramedics are bringing Yumi to the hospital. Stevens tells Bailey, "She collapsed at the Taste of Seattle and is vomiting blood." Bailey replies, "Damn fool, probably tore her esophagus in two by now." Yumi has emergency surgery to repair the extensive damage. In the recovery room, Mr. Kamaji tells intern Dr. Karev, "I thought she would be fine. I'm sorry." Karev informs Kamaji of the consequences of pushing Yumi to compete that afternoon, saying, "Don't tell me. Tell her. Tell her how her career is over because of you."

Health professionals criticize patients who did not follow mainstream medicine practices. For example, in the *House, M.D.* pilot,[50] the mother admits that she has not been giving her asthmatic son his inhaler as prescribed because, she says, "I worry about children taking such strong medicine so frequently." House lectures the woman on not listening to the doctor and then dismisses the woman, saying, "Forget it. If you don't trust steroids, you shouldn't trust doctors." In "I Do"[51] of *ER*, doctors diagnose a boy with AIDS-related pneumonia and then learn that his mother did not protect her children in the womb or have them tested after birth because she believes that AIDS is not a disease, but a conspiracy. Dr. Clemente criticizes the woman, stating, "She knew she was infected and she did nothing to protect her child. It's the most moronic, selfish..." After Clemente leaves, a nurse begs the mother to allow treatment, "If you let this go on like this, there's not going to be a doctor that can help him. He only has you." The mother agrees to treat her son, but refuses to let the medical staff test or treat her other child for HIV.

Doctors also criticize people who chose not to vaccinate because they had read literature on the dangers of immunizations. For example, in the *House, M.D.* episode "Paternity,"[52] a young mother tells House that she is not vaccinating her baby. House asks her, "You don't think they work?" She responds, "I think some multinational pharmaceutical company wants me to think they work. Pad their bottom line." House lectures her on her misguided beliefs:

House: The antibodies in yummy mummy only protect the kid for six months, which is why these companies think they can gouge you. They think that you'll spend whatever they ask to keep your kid alive. Want to change things? Prove them wrong. A few hundred parents like you decide they'd rather let their kid die than cough up 40 bucks for a vaccination, believe me, prices will drop REALLY fast.

House then diagnoses the baby with a cold.

In the *ER* episode "A Walk in the Woods,"[53] the consequences of a parent's decision to not vaccinate her son are much more severe. A woman tells doctors that she did not have her son immunized because of the risk of autism. Doctors diagnose the boy with measles. In the course of the episode, the boy stops breathing and dies, demonstrating that the risks of not vaccinating can be far worse than the risks of the immunizations. Such stories are reflected in real-life consequences. For example, David Sugarman and colleagues found a 2008 measles outbreak was geographically clustered around communities with intentionally unvaccinated and under-vaccinated children.[54] Given the implications for those who cannot be immunized, this trend toward vaccine refusal is especially alarming.

Most episodes portray the doctor-patient-parent relationships as paternalistic, in which patients blindly trusted and accepted the opinions of their physicians. It was unusual for patients to choose alternative health practices, propose their own diagnosis or treatment or question the physicians. These findings reflect traditional representations of the heroic, infallible physician.[55] Given that these dramas rely on real-life physicians for storylines and issues with accuracy, the positive depictions are not surprising. However, this heroic doctor representation discourages active patients: why question doctors' decisions when they are always right?

With the trend toward the active patient, one would expect more fictional storylines that present the doctor-patient relationship as a partnership. Physicians criticized patients who argued with them or discussed research they had done about their health. These reactions may discourage people from asking questions or from voicing their opinions. If patients believe that their doctors will ignore their questions or become irritated, they may be less likely to ask them. This finding is not unique to fictional television. In real-life, many doctors believe patients' questions about online material wastes their time, and are therefore, unnecessary.[56] This message contradicts contemporary literature on improving patient care, discouraging people from taking active roles in their health care. In more positive portrayals, fictional doctors could be receptive to patient questions, indirectly informing viewers on deciphering between credible and false information.[57] These programs could also discuss online support groups or other resources for people seeking additional health knowledge.

Attempts at self-treating caused ill health for many fictional patients. And yet, it is not feasible or cost-efficient for people to seek medical care for every minor injury or simple illness. Storylines could educate viewers by introducing remedies for common ailments. For example, in *ER* and *Grey's Anatomy*, Drs. Corday, Greene, and Montgomery develop poison ivy reactions. These cases could have addressed home remedies, such as calamine lotion or oatmeal baths.

Practices outside of mainstream medicine resulted in dire consequences for patients. Overall, these dramas presented a dichotomy between mainstream and alternative health practices. In reality, many benefits exist for combining the two. Increasingly, physicians and other health professionals are recognizing the value of using homeopathic medicine to supplement mainstream care.[58] For example, a patient with a urinary tract infection (UTI) may take prescribed antibiotics and a cranberry supplement to cure the infection and reduce the risk of further attacks.[59] Complementary or alternative treatments are often administered along with conventional medicine for chronic conditions or disease, such as multiple sclerosis or breast cancer.[60] Storylines could also highlight the benefits of alternative health choices, teaching people the benefits of combining homeopathic medicine with mainstream medicine and including common home remedies.

For health choices that are not supported by mainstream medicine, these programs could include more information to support their positions. Similar to real-life cases, doctors were dismissive (at the very least) of families who refused to vaccinate.[61] The pro-immunization messages were not surprising since *ER* was part of a public health campaign to encourage vaccination.[62] However, these programs did little to educate people about vaccine safety or other issues that may improve immunization rates. Instead of only criticism, a more positive approach would model open communication about vaccinations.[63] Discussions of herd immunity, for example, may help parents conceptualize immunization as a public health responsibility, instead of a private choice.[64] Research has shown that these conversations are important to maintaining trust between doctors and families who refuse to vaccinate.[65] These conversations could also help viewers who are uncertain about their immunization decisions.

CONCLUSION

Even with non-preventable conditions, patients are constructed as responsible for their ill health in medical dramas. Fictional health professionals blame patients for failing to follow their advice and poorly managing chronic conditions. Furthermore, patients are criticized or even face negative health consequences when they exhibit characters of an "active" patient, by asking questions, seeking information online, and requesting a second opinion. Throughout these programs, medical dramas hold individual patients responsible for needing care, missing storyline opportunities to educate viewers about when to seek treatment, how to research credible medical information, the importance of second opinions, and the proper means of managing chronic conditions. In addition, entertainment television ignores real-life shifts in the doctor-patient relationship, instead perpetuating an outdated paternalistic approach to care, in which patients silently accept diagnosis and treatment, rather than share in the decision-making process. Since extensive research has established that medical dramas model this relationship, regardless of how realistic the portrayals may be, these programs teach viewers to stay quiet and not question, as opposed to the engaged approach recommended in patient safety literature. Finally, these representations discourage one to partake in some of the alternative health choices that may reduce the need for prescription medicine or visits to one's health provider. Given that most people routinely use the Internet for information, this representation is not realistic, nor ideal for quality patient care.

NOTES

1. Shore, *The Trust Crisis in Health care*.
2. Emanuel and Emanuel, "Four Models of the Physician-Patient Relationship."
3. Tu and Cohen, "Striking Jump in Consumers Seeking Health Care Information."
4. Ibid.; Murray, E. et al., "The Impact of Health Information on the Internet on the Physician-Patient Relationship."
5. Murray, E. et al., "The Impact of Health Information on the Internet on the Physician-Patient Relationship"; Iverson, Howard, and Penney, "Impact of Internet Use on Health-Related Behaviors and the Patient-Physician Relationship"; Epstein, R.M., Alper, B.S., and Quill, T.E., "Communicating Evidence for Participatory Decision Making."
6. Berger, Wagner, and Baker, "Internet Use and Stigmatized Illness."
7. Bergeson, S.C., and Dean, J.D., "A Systems Approach to Patient-Centered Care."
8. Flanagan-Klygis, E.A., Sharp, L., and Frader, J.E., "Dismissing the Family Who Refuses Vaccines."
9. Marvel, M. et al., "Soliciting the Patient's Agenda."
10. Ahmad et al., "Are Physicians Ready for Patients With Internet-Based Health Information?".
11. Ibid.; Crocco, A.G., Villasis-Keever, M., and Jadad, A.R., "Analysis of Cases of Harm Associated with Use of Health Information on the Internet"; Peterson and Fretz, "Patient Use of the Internet for Information in a Lung Cancer Clinic*."
12. Ahmad et al., "Are Physicians Ready for Patients With Internet-Based Health Information?"; Hardey, "Doctor in the House."
13. "Patients Doubt Doctors' Advice When It Conflicts With Online Info - iHealthBeat."
14. Murray, E. et al., "The Impact of Health Information on the Internet on the Physician-Patient Relationship."
15. Albert, *Wake Up*.
16. Chulack, *Man With No Name*.
17. Glatter, *Let It Be*.
18. Moore, *Let the Games Begin*.
19. O'Fallon, *TB or Not TB*.
20. Marvel, M. et al., "Soliciting the Patient's Agenda."

21. Ibid.

22. Muzio, *Refusal of Care*.

23. Sharf and Freimuth, "The Construction of Illness on Entertainment Television."

24. Scott, *Genevieve and the Fat Boy*.

25. "Second Opinions: Greater Understanding."

26. Chulack, *Exodus*.

27. Kaplan, *A Shot in the Dark*.

28. Alcala, *Safe*.

29. Briggs et al., "The Role of Specialist Neuroradiology Second Opinion Reporting"; Morrow, M. et al., "Surgeon Recommendations and Receipt of Mastectomy for Treatment of Breast Cancer."

30. "Second Surgical Opinions."

31. Kaplan, *Orion in the Sky*.

32. Chulack, *Rescue Me*.

33. Chaudhary, Solomon, and Cosgrove, "The Relationship between Perceived Risk of Being Ticketed and Self-Reported Seat Belt Use."

34. "CDC - Chronic Disease - Overview."

35. Ibid.

36. Ibid.

37. Mann, *Don't Stand So Close to Me*.

38. "CDC - Diabetes Statistics and Research - Diabetes & Me - Diabetes DDT."

39. Misiano, *Great Expectations*.

40. Holcomb, *Last Call*.

41. *Vanishing Act*.

42. Trevino, *Second Chances*.

43. Morgan et al., "In Their Own Words."

44. "Organdonor.gov | The Need Is Real."

45. *Insurrection*.

46. Sarafian, *Autopsy*.

47. "Trends in In-Hospital Newborn Male Circumcision —— United States, 1999–2010."

48. Robinson, *Band Aid Covers the Bullet Hole*.

49. *Tell Me Sweet Little Lies*.

50. Singer, *Pilot*.

51. Muzio, *I Do*.

52. O'Fallon, *Paternity*.

53. Wells, *A Walk in the Woods*."

54. Sugerman et al., "Measles Outbreak in a Highly Vaccinated Population, San Diego, 2008."

55. Turow, *Playing Doctor*; Jacobs, *Body Trauma TV*.

56. Ahmad et al., "Are Physicians Ready for Patients With Internet-Based Health Information?"

57. Crocco, A.G., Villasis-Keever, M., and Jadad, A.R., "Analysis of Cases of Harm Associated with Use of Health Information on the Internet."

58. Astin, J.A. et al., "A Review of the Incorporation of Complementary and Alternative Medicine by Mainstream Physicians."

59. Jepson, Mihaljevic, and Craig, "Cranberries for Preventing Urinary Tract Infections."

60. Berkman et al., "Use of Alternative Treatments by People with Multiple Sclerosis"; Shen et al., "Use of Complementary/alternative Therapies by Women with Advanced-Stage Breast Cancer."

61. Flanagan-Klygis, E.A., Sharp, L., and Frader, J.E., "Dismissing the Family Who Refuses Vaccines."

62. Glik et al., "Health Education Goes Hollywood."

63. Leask et al., "Communicating with Parents about Vaccination."

64. Pe, "Herd Immunity."

65. Fortune and Wilson, "Preserving Relationships with Antivaccine Parents Five Suggestions from Social Psychology."

Chapter Seven

Beyond Medical Dramas

Connecting Media to Contemporary Health Care

After forty years of the personal responsibility model, where is medicine at now? Improved diagnostic tools and treatments have helped decrease cancer-related deaths by 20 percent.[1] The development of antiretroviral therapy has enabled people with HIV to live for decades after diagnosis.[2] We can contain many outbreaks before they become pandemics, as demonstrated with Severe Acute Respiratory Syndrome (SARS).[3] Scientists can map DNA, understanding the makeup of the human genome.[4] Diseases that plagued humans for centuries are no longer on our radar or even part of our collective memory, as evidenced by the increase in non-medical immunizations.[5]

At the same time, "modern medicine" has yet to cure all of society's ailments. Although some strides have made toward cell regeneration, we still cannot adequately treat spinal cord injuries.[6] An estimated 60–70 million Americans live with bowel and digestive disorders, generating over $100 billion in medical expenses each year.[7] It is beyond the reach of doctors to halt many devastating degenerative diseases, like muscular dystrophy or multiple sclerosis.[8] Life expectancy is still at 78.7 years, hardly a change from 30 years ago, with 74.6 years for the average person.[9] For perspective, from 1900 to 1959, the life expectancy rose 20 years.[10]

As we have known since the 1970s, living longer often means living with chronic illnesses that include heart disease, diabetes, cancer, stroke, arthritis, osteoporosis, and other debilitating conditions, many of which will ultimately kill us.[11] With all our knowledge about prevention, as a society, we haven't fared very well. Despite the extensive campaigns educating people on healthy behaviors, Americans continue to smoke, excessively drink, text and drive, consume junk food, and spend far too much time on the couch.

Even with America's obsession with appearance, fueled by reality makeover shows and skeleton-like models, the obesity rate in America is at an all-time high, with over a third of adults and 18 percent of children considered obese.[12] Approximately 75 percent of health care costs can be attributed to chronic diseases, including type 2 diabetes, cardiovascular disease, and other conditions, many of which all can be controlled or even prevented with healthy lifestyles.[13]

What behaviors have we successfully modified? Seat belt usage has increased significantly, from 11 percent in 1980 to 1990, with approximately 85 percent of American drivers buckling up.[14] This change can largely be attributed to financial penalties, conveyed through the "Click It or Ticket" campaign.[15] Reye Syndrome, caused by giving children aspirin, has been almost entirely eliminated.[16] Fewer people are drinking and driving, thanks to the Designated Driver campaign, paired with steep fines for this behavior.[17] From these effective campaigns, we know that Americans can and will adopt healthy behaviors if a suitable alternative is available (i.e., giving Tylenol, instead of aspirin), people perceive themselves at risk, and the negative consequences outweigh the pleasure of the behavior, such as the fines for no seatbelts.

Campaigns are far less effective without clear, immediate incentives for changing the behavior. Recent legislation, including the Patient Protection and Affordable Care Act (ACA), is designed to create a climate of success for healthy behavior. For example, public smoking bans have been much more effective in curbing smoking than years of anti-tobacco messages.[18] Likewise, employee wellness programs have yielded great success in reducing health risks for participants.[19] The free preventative care mandated by ACA is likely going to encourage well check-ups, mammograms, and immunizations much more than public health advocates lecturing on the importance of these actions, without offering a means to pay for them.

Yet, many Americans have ardently opposed any legislation that impacts individual behavior, even if that behavior will likely lead to an early death. At least some of this can be explained through the American desire for individual choices. As Starr outlined, government intervention is necessary to keep America running smoothly.[20] Without government-run programs, we would not have Social Security, public education, parks, or other aspects of life that organize society, which also include mandated insurance, caps on hospital bills, the elimination of pre-existing conditions for insurance enrollment, preventative care and wellness programs.

People also question the Patient Safety Movement, fearing that it will hinder the autonomy of health professionals—the same autonomy that has led to a culture of medical errors. While some action has been taken to reduce mistakes, many of the problems identified in the IOM reports still exist.[21] Errors due to medication, misdiagnosis, delayed diagnosis, treatment, and miscommunication still occur.[22] Even with literature that demonstrates the importance of open communication, not all health professionals support the disclosure of medical errors.[23] In addition, while the publicity about medical errors led to "Sign Your Site" and other programs aimed to decrease errors, this attention also exacerbated health professionals' fear of malpractice.[24] As a result, some health care providers have become overly cautious, ordering unnecessary tests or performing unnecessary surgery to protect against perceptions of medical mistakes.[25] Such actions are costly and can impact overall patient care—for example, prompting physicians to perform cesarean sections as a precaution to complications.[26]

Why do we hold fast to individualism at the expense of our national health? America prides itself on choice, even when it can lead to self-destruction, as exemplified by the housing crisis of the mid-2000s, when numerous people bought houses they could not afford leading to massive foreclosures. It does not help that health care reform often conflicts with other messages that celebrate individualism, choice, and the American Dream in news and entertainment media. The rogue TV doc that breaks protocol is usually considered a hero. Few television storylines address insurance, bureaucracy, or other macro issues that are a daily reality of real-life health care. From these programs, media consumers receive contradictory messages about health responsibility as patients. On one hand, public health discourse advises people to take charge of their health, an approach paired with wellness incentives. Yet, entertainment television mocks "active patients," often with dire consequences for those who treat themselves or question their health care provider. Such resistance on-screen is rooted in real-life opposition to patient participation, as indicated by surveys of physicians who discourage patients from researching their medical conditions.[27]

Obviously, the discussion here has been focused on one genre: medical dramas. While these programs have consistently been a part of television since the early 1950s, the representations here are not the only media source influencing perceptions of health professionals and patients. Exploring other media products produce similar themes of individualism, the paradox of the flawed and heroic doctors and the conflicting messages about personal responsibility, mixed with attacks of the overzealous patient.

The personally flawed, skilled health professional prevail in sitcoms, with the quirky cast of *Scrubs*, and more recently, Mindy Kaling as Dr. Lahiri in *The Mindy Project*. Reminiscent of *M*A*S*H**, these docs humorously struggle with basic life tasks and relationships, but treat and cure their patients with ease. At the same time, the popularity of crime dramas in the 2000s has perpetuated a much darker image of the TV doc. In this genre, doctors and nurses usually appear in guest roles as unscrupulous villains. For example, a physician character conducts twisted Dr. Moreau-esque experiments in the *CSI: Crime Scene Investigation* episode "Pirates of the Third

Reich,"[28] physically sewing together two men, killing them in the process. Similarly, in "God Complex"[29] of *Criminal Minds*, a serial killer amputates healthy limbs of his victims and then reattaches them to other people. And in *American Horror Story*, a psychiatrist severs the legs of a patient to prevent her from escaping in "Nor'easter."[30] As with the few flawed guest docs in medical dramas, these villains appear in a single episode and are caught and punished by the authorities/protagonists of the programs (i.e., CSIs, F.B.I. profilers, and detectives).

Legal dramas have conveyed tamer, but still disturbing portrayals of fictional health professionals. They appear as expert witnesses or, sometimes, as criminals, usually because of medical-related breach of ethics. For example, in the *Law & Order: SVU* episode "Starved,"[31] a surgeon rapes women he meets through a dating service. The episode evolved into an ethical debate about assisted suicide. Law programs have also run storylines with doctors as the victims of crime, often related to their medical specialties. For example, in the *Law & Order: Special Victims Unit* episode "Silencer,"[32] an ear surgeon is murdered because he performed cochlear implant surgeries (a device that improves hearing). The detectives determine that deaf activists killed him as a protest to the surgeries themselves—fictionalizing heated real-life cochlear implant debates. Like crime dramas, these doctor characters only exist for an episode or two to support the main protagonists' investigation. And the focus is on the individual doctors, not the health care system as a whole.

In other types of dramas, physicians are representative of the "establishment" or corrupt authority figures that govern the protagonists. In the Netflix original prison drama, *Orange is the New Black*, the female inmates constantly battle the guards, pharmacist, and prison doctors for health tools that maintain quality of life. For example, Sophia, a transgendered inmate, fights for months to receive the appropriate hormone dosage after a prison physician takes her off the medication, disregarding the dire impact on Sophia's health. Similarly, the prisoners fear the Psych ward, which keeps its patients so heavily medicated that few are allowed to return to minimal security. In this program, health professionals play minor roles, only appearing in occasional episodes. Their actions reinforce the recurrent struggle that the prisoners survive their sentences without too much irreparable damage to mental and physical health.

We also see individualism perpetuated through the actions of regular characters in a health crisis, particularly with supernatural shows, which highlight and reward self-sufficiency. The premise of the postmodern drama *Lost* demands survival tactics. On an island, with few supplies, survivors either make do or perish, particularly in the early episodes of the show. For example, in the pilot episode, a survivor without medical training easily learns how to suture a wound.[33] Likewise, the post-apocalyptic zombie drama, *The Walking Dead*, celebrates resourcefulness. Those that persist through the endless feeding-frenzies of the "walkers" are brave, independent and tough, as exemplified with the cowboy protagonist Rick, or are protected by these types of characters. In this show, characters are surprisingly successful at treating zombie and non-zombie inflicted maladies, with people surviving gunshot wounds, blood poisoning, amputations, disease, and other injuries that would be life-threatening even if treated in a hospital. In season one, for example, the character Merle severs his own hand with a hacksaw and cauterizes the wound, while fending off a herd of walkers. He survives for three seasons before he is finally killed—not by "walkers," but a gunshot to the head. When a flu-like epidemic sweeps through the prison camp in season four, most survive, despite the close quarters and harsh conditions, aided by Hershel, a retired veterinarian. Each episode rewards individual actions situated in a world without government or other institutions.

The popularity of reality television in the 2000s took self-sufficiency to a whole new level, showcasing what "regular" people are capable of, with very little professional guidance. Dislike your current floor plan? The crew of *Trading Spaces* taught you to take a sledgehammer and knock down a wall. Find yourself stranded in the desert? Bear Grylls (in *Man vs. Wild*) showed us how to turn a rattlesnake into a makeshift canteen, filled with one's own urine. This genre has included a wealth of advice for health improvement as well, from superficial physical upgrades in *What Not to Wear* to *The Biggest Loser* guiding viewers on weight loss. With this genre came a slew of shows highlighting the dangers of medical errors. Fitting with the rise of the Patient Safety Movement, shows on The Learning Channel (TLC) and Discovery Health, warned viewers of the prevalence of medical errors. For example, each episode of the program *Mystery Diagnosis* (2005–present) features multiple patients' stories of misdiagnosis. People recall to the camera how they became progressively sicker, yet doctors either did not believe them or could not cure them. In the show's resolution, patients stumble onto qualified care providers who solve the "mystery." Overall, this program perpetuates distrust and incompetency in the health profession. Likewise, the self-explanatory titles of *When Surgical Tools Get Left Behind: 1 and 2* convey similar messages of ineptitude, blaming individuals for forgetting scissors, sponges and other objects inside patients' surgical wounds. In all of these programs, most of the health professionals appear callous and incompetent, save the final doc who determines the correct diagnosis and treatment. Little is said about the flaws in the system or recent macro changes that help decrease errors. While 1500 foreign objects per year are left behind in patients, in recent years, instrument counts and other preventative protocol have been implemented.[34] These actions demonstrate systematic problems, not individual ones, largely cause errors, despite public discourse that says otherwise.

Why has television presented a distorted picture of doctors, patients, and the overall health profession? Michael Crichton wrote the original script for *ER* (debuting in 1994) in the 1970s.[35] Would viewers have been interested in a real-life picture of health care, with its mountains of paperwork, hours of waiting, and mundane cases of strep throat and chest pain? Perhaps realistic medicine is simply too dull for television, in the way that a realistic crime show would bore viewers to tears as they painstakingly watched Crime Scene Investigators wait weeks or even months for DNA results on a cotton swab (without the jazzy montage)? But this approach is problematic, setting viewers up for disappointment at their next visits. We know that people learn about medicine from television, from specific diseases and treatments, to information gleaned about the process of health care.[36] Audience members largely believe these shows, despite their known inaccuracies and exaggerations.[37] We are taught how we should act as patients, when we should seek a second opinion, and what a "doctor" looks like from entertainment television.[38] The messages then, that herald individual doctors as heroes and demonize those that err as "bad apples" have contributed to our resistance of macro change in the health care system. An ideological shield has been created, convincing us that an individual's actions (doctor or patient) determines good health care experiences and health overall.

The knowledge, that television informs consumers and influences behavior, could better be used to garner support for health care reform. More news and entertainment media messages that clarify health care policies, showcase the benefits of this legislation and reinforce the necessity of an insured population would help correct current myths and misperceptions about sacrificing individual freedom for the common good. At this point, as the glitches of implementing a new system are still being worked out, it is unclear how the Patient Safety movement and the Affordable Care Act will truly change health care in the United States. Will the government absorb the overall responsibility for preventing medical errors and improving health? How can we advocate health prevention, without assigning blame for "preventable" conditions? Are Americans capable of sacrificing a small percentage of individual choice in exchange for better overall health? Good or bad, the media, as a primary institution in America will help us navigate this new approach to health care.

NOTES

1. Siegel et al., "Cancer Statistics, 2014."
2. Samji et al., "Closing the Gap."
3. Disease, "CDC - SARS - Basics Fact Sheet."
4. Collins et al., "New Goals for the U.S. Human Genome Project."
5. Omer, S.B. et al., "Nonmedical Exemptions to School Immunization Requirements."

6. Office of Communications and Public Liaison, "Spinal Cord Injury: Hope Through Research."

7. National Institutes of Health, *Opportunities and Challenges in Digestive Diseases Research: Recommendations of the National Commission on Digestive Diseases.*

8. Board, "Muscular Dystrophy"; "Multiple Sclerosis."

9. Arias, "United States Life Tables, 2008."

10. Ibid.

11. "CDC - Chronic Disease - Overview."

12. Ogden et al., "Prevalence of Obesity in the United States, 2009–2010"; "CDC - Obesity - Facts - Adolescent and School Health."

13. "CDC - Chronic Disease - At A Glance."

14. *Increased Safety-Belt Use—United States, 1991*; "CDC."

15. Chaudhary, Solomon, and Cosgrove, "The Relationship between Perceived Risk of Being Ticketed and Self-Reported Seat Belt Use."

16. Soumerai, Ross-Degnan, and Kahn, "The Effects of Professional and Media Warnings About the Association Between aspirin Use in Children and Reye's Syndrome."

17. Winsten, "Promoting Designated Drivers."

18. "Smoking Bans Cut Number of Heart Attacks, Strokes."

19. Berry, Mirabito, and Baun, *What's the Hard Return on Employee Wellness Programs?*.

20. Starr, *Remedy and Reaction.*

21. America et al., *To Err Is Human.*

22. Pham et al., "Reducing Medical Errors and Adverse Events."

23. Iezzoni et al., "Survey Shows That At Least Some Physicians Are Not Always Open Or Honest With Patients."

24. Baker, *The Medical Malpractice Myth.*

25. Studdert, D.M. et al., "Defensive Medicine among High-Risk Specialist Physicians in a Volatile Malpractice Environment."

26. Baker, *The Medical Malpractice Myth.*

27. Ahmad et al., "Are Physicians Ready for Patients With Internet-Based Health Information?"; Bergeson, S.C. and Dean, J.D., "A Systems Approach to Patient-Centered Care."

28. Lewis, *Pirates of the Third Reich.*

29. Teng, *God Complex.*

30. Uppendahl, *Nor'easter.*

31. Platt, *Starved.*

32. White, *Silencer.*

33. Abrams, *Pilot.*

34. Whang et al., "Left Behind"; "Surgical Implements Too Often Left Behind in Patients."

35. Turow, *Playing Doctor.*

36. Glik et al., "Health Education Goes Hollywood"; Gauthier, "Television Drama and Popular Film as Medical Narrative"; Turow, "Television Entertainment and the US Health-Care Debate."

37. Baer, "Cardiopulmonary Resuscitation on Television. Exaggerations and Accusations"; Davin, "Healthy Viewing: The Reception of Medical Narratives."

38. Turow, "Television Entertainment and the US Health-Care Debate"; Gauthier, "Television Drama and Popular Film as Medical Narrative."

Bibliography

01, Jul, and 2000. "Issues in the 2000 Election: Health Care." Accessed January 16, 2014. http://kff.org/uninsured/poll-finding/issues-in-the-2000-election-health-care/.

"20 Tips to Help Prevent Medical Errors." Text, September 1, 2011. http://www.ahrq.gov/patients-consumers/care-planning/errors/20tips/index.html.

30, Apr, and 2013. "Kaiser Health Tracking Poll: April 2013." Accessed January 16, 2014. http://kff.org/health-reform/poll-finding/kaiser-health-tracking-poll-april-2013/.

Abrams, J. J. *Pilot*. Television program. Lost. Bad Robot, 2004.

Ahmad, Farah, Pamela L Hudak, Kim Bercovitz, Elisa Hollenberg, and Wendy Levinson. "Are Physicians Ready for Patients With Internet-Based Health Information?" *Journal of Medical Internet Research* 8, no. 3 (September 29, 2006). doi:10.2196/jmir.8.3.e22.

Albert, Arthur. *Wake Up*. Television program. ER. Warner Brothers, 2005.

Alcala, Felix Enriquez. *Safe*. Television program. House, M.D. Bad Hat Harry Productions, 2006.

Allegrante, J.P., and L.W. Green. "Sounding Board. When Health Policy Becomes Victim Blaming." *The New England Journal of Medicine* 305, no. 25 (December 17, 1981): 1528–1529. doi:10.1056/NEJM198112173052511.

America, Committee on Quality of Health Care in, Institute of Medicine, Linda T. Kohn, Janet M. Corrigan, and Molla S. Donaldson. *To Err Is Human: Building a Safer Health System*. 1st edition. National Academies Press, 2000.

Anderson, Ann. *Snake Oil, Hustlers and Hambones: The American Medicine Show*. McFarland, 2004.

Annas, G J. "Reframing the Debate on Health Care Reform by Replacing Our Metaphors." *The New England Journal of Medicine* 332, no. 11 (March 16, 1995): 744–47.

Annas, George J. "Sex, Money, and Bioethics Watching ER and Chicago Hope." *Hastings Center Report* 25, no. 5 (1995): 40–43. doi:10.2307/3562794.

Arias, Elizabeth. "United States Life Tables, 2008." *National Vital Statistics Reports* 61, no. 3 (September 24, 2012): 1–64.

Astin, J.A., Marie, A., Pelletier, K.R., Hansen, E., and Haskell, W.L. "A Review of the Incorporation of Complementary and Alternative Medicine by Mainstream Physicians." *Archives of Internal Medicine* 158, no. 21 (November 23, 1998): 2303–2310. doi:10.1001/archinte.158.21.2303.

Baer, N.A. "Cardiopulmonary Resuscitation on Television. Exaggerations and Accusations." *The New England Journal of Medicine* 334, no. 24 (June 13, 1996): 1604–1605. doi:10.1056/NEJM199606133342412.

Baker, Tom. *The Medical Malpractice Myth*. Chicago: University of Chicago Press, 2007.

Barry, John M. *The Great Influenza: The Story of the Deadliest Plague in History*. New York: Penguin Books, 2005.

Basil, Michael D. "Identification as a Mediator of Celebrity Effects." *Journal of Broadcasting & Electronic Media* 40, no. 4 (1996): 478–95. doi:10.1080/08838159609364370.

Bauer, Jeffrey C., Healthcare Financial Management Association (U.S.), and Educational Foundation. *Not What the Doctor Ordered: How to End the Medical Monopoly in Pursuit of Managed Care*. New York: McGraw-Hill, 1998.

Bellah, Robert N. *Habits of the Heart: Individualism and Commitment in American Life : With a New Preface*. Berkeley: University of California Press, 2008.

Bennfield, Robert L. *Who Loses Coverage for How Long?* Current Population Reports. Household Economic Studies, May 1996. http://www.census.gov/sipp/p70-54.pdf.

Berg, Frances M. *Underage and Overweight: America's Childhood Obesity Crisis - What Every Parent Needs to Know*. New York, NY: Hatherleigh Press, 2004.

Berger, Magdalena, Todd H. Wagner, and Laurence C. Baker. "Internet Use and Stigmatized Illness." *Social Science & Medicine* 61, no. 8 (October 2005): 1821–1827. doi:10.1016/j.socscimed.2005.03.025.

Berger, Peter L, and Thomas Luckmann. *The Social Construction of Reality: A Treatise in the Sociology of Knowledge*. Garden City, N.Y.: Doubleday, 1967.

Bergeson, S.C., and Dean, J.D. "A Systems Approach to Patient-Centered Care." *JAMA* 296, no. 23 (December 20, 2006): 2848–2851. doi:10.1001/jama.296.23.2848.

Berkman, Cathy S., Monica G. Pignotti, Pamela F. Cavallo, and Nancy J. Holland. "Use of Alternative Treatments by People with Multiple Sclerosis." *Neurorehabilitation and Neural Repair* 13, no. 4 (December 1, 1999): 243–254. doi:10.1177/154596839901300406.

Berry, Leonard, Ann M. Mirabito, and William B. Baun. *What's the Hard Return on Employee Wellness Programs?* SSRN Scholarly Paper. Rochester, NY: Social Science Research Network, 2010. http://papers.ssrn.com/abstract=2064874.

Bishop, Gene, and Amy C. Brodkey. "Personal Responsibility and Physician Responsibility — West Virginia's Medicaid Plan." *New England Journal of Medicine* 355, no. 8 (2006): 756–758. doi:10.1056/NEJMp068170.

Blendon, Robert J., Catherine M. DesRoches, Mollyann Brodie, John M. Benson, Allison B. Rosen, Eric Schneider, Drew E. Altman, Kinga Zapert, Melissa J. Herrmann, and Annie E. Steffenson. "Views of Practicing Physicians and the Public on Medical Errors." *New England Journal of Medicine* 347, no. 24 (2002): 1933–1940. doi:10.1056/NEJMsa022151.

Blendon, Robert. "Why Americans Don't Trust the Government and Don't Trust Healthcare." In *The Trust Crisis in Healthcare*, edited by David A. Shore, 21–31. Oxford; New York: Oxford University Press, 2007.

Blumenfeld, William. "Some Correlates of TV Medical Drama Viewing." *Psychological Reports* 15 (1964): 901–2.

Board, A. D. A. M. Editorial. "Muscular Dystrophy." Text, February 1, 2012. http://www.ncbi.nlm.nih.gov/pubmedhealth/PMH0002172/.

Briggs, G. M., P. A. Flynn, M. Worthington, I. Rennie, and C. S. McKinstry. "The Role of Specialist Neuroradiology Second Opinion Reporting: Is There Added Value?" *Clinical Radiology* 63, no. 7 (July 2008): 791–795. doi:10.1016/j.crad.2007.12.002.

Brodie, Mollyann, Ursula Foehr, Vicky Rideout, Neal Baer, Carolyn Miller, Rebecca Flournoy, and Drew Altman. "Communicating Health Information Through The Entertainment Media." *Health Affairs* 20, no. 1 (January 1, 2001): 192–99. doi:10.1377/hlthaff.20.1.192.

Brownmiller, Susan. *Against Our Will: Men, Women, and Rape*. New York: Fawcett Books, 1993.

Burnham, John. "American Medicine's Golden Age: What Happened to It?" *Science* 2115, no. 4539 (1982): 1474–79.

Butler, Nattinger A., Hoffmann, R.G., Howell-Pelz, A., and Goodwin, J.S. "Effect of Nancy Reagan's Mastectomy on Choice of Surgery for Breast Cancer by US Women." *JAMA* 279, no. 10 (March 11, 1998): 762–66. doi:10.1001/jama.279.10.762.

Campbell, Jr., Darrell, A., and Patricia, L. Cornett. "How Stress and Burnout Produce Medical Mistakes." In *Medical Error: What Do We Know? What Do We Do?*, edited by Marilynn M.

Rosenthal and Kathleen M Sutcliffe, 37–57. San Francisco, Calif.: Jossey-Bass Publishers, 2006.

Carey, James W. *Communication as Culture: Essays on Media and Society*. New York (N.Y.) [etc.]: Routledge, 1989.

Cassedy, James H. *Medicine in America: A Short History*. Baltimore: Johns Hopkins University Press, 1991.

"CDC - Chronic Disease - At A Glance." Accessed January 15, 2014. http://www.cdc.gov/chronicdisease/resources/publications/AAG/chronic.htm.

"CDC - Chronic Disease - Overview." Accessed January 15, 2014. http://www.cdc.gov/chronicdisease/overview/index.htm.

"CDC - Diabetes Statistics and Research - Diabetes & Me - Diabetes DDT." Accessed January 16, 2014. http://www.cdc.gov/diabetes/consumer/research.htm.

"CDC - Fact Sheets-Alcohol Use and Health - Alcohol." Accessed January 15, 2014. http://www.cdc.gov/alcohol/fact-sheets/alcohol-use.htm.

"CDC - Obesity - Facts - Adolescent and School Health." Accessed January 15, 2014. http://www.cdc.gov/HealthyYouth/obesity/facts.htm.

"CDC: Seat Belt Use Reaches 85 Percent." Accessed January 15, 2014. http://phys.org/news/2011-01-cdc-seat-belt-percent.html.

Chaudhary, Neil K., Mark G. Solomon, and Linda A. Cosgrove. "The Relationship between Perceived Risk of Being Ticketed and Self-Reported Seat Belt Use." *Journal of Safety Research* 35, no. 4 (2004): 383–390. doi:10.1016/j.jsr.2004.03.015.

Chory-Assad, Rebecca M., and Ron Tamborini. "Television Doctors: An Analysis of Physicians in Fictional and Non-Fictional Television Programs." *Journal of Broadcasting & Electronic Media* 45, no. 3 (2001): 499–521. doi:10.1207/s15506878jobem4503_8.

———. "Television Exposure and the Public's Perceptions of Physicians." *Journal of Broadcasting & Electronic Media* 47, no. 2 (2003): 197–215. doi:10.1207/s15506878jobem4702_3.

Chulack, Christopher. *Exodus*. Television program. ER. Warner Brothers, 1998.

———. *Man With No Name*. Television program. ER. Warner Brothers, 2005.

———. *Rescue Me*. Television program. Warner Brothers, 2000.

Clarke, Juanne N. "Cancer, Heart Disease, and AIDS: What Do The Media Tell Us About These Diseases?" *Health Communication* 4, no. 2 (1992): 105–20. doi:10.1207/s15327027hc0402_2.

Cohen, Marc R., and Audrey Shafer. "Images and Healers: A Visual History of Scientific Medicine." In *Cultural Sutures: Medicine and Media*, 197–214. Durham, N.C.: Duke University Press, 2004.

Collins, Francis S., Ari Patrinos, Elke Jordan, Aravinda Chakravarti, Raymond Gesteland, and LeRoy Walters. "New Goals for the U.S. Human Genome Project: 1998–2003." *Science* 282, no. 5389 (October 23, 1998): 682–689. doi:10.1126/science.282.5389.682.

Crane, Diana. *The Sociology of Culture: Emerging Theoretical Perspectives*. Oxford [etc.]: Blackwell, 1994.

Crichton, Michael. *Dr. Carter, I Presume*. Television program. ER. Warner Brothers, 1996.

———. *Forgive and Forget*. Television program. ER. Warner Brothers, 2004.

———. *Out of Africa*. Television program. ER. Warner Brothers, 2003.

———. *Sharp Relief*. Television program. ER. Warner Brothers, 1998.

———. *Time of Death*. Television program. ER. Warner Brothers, 2004.

Crocco, A.G., Villasis-Keever, M., and Jadad, A.R. "Analysis of Cases of Harm Associated with Use of Health Information on the Internet." *JAMA* 287, no. 21 (June 5, 2002): 2869–2871. doi:10.1001/jama.287.21.2869.

Davin, Solange. "Healthy Viewing: The Reception of Medical Narratives." In *Health and the Media*, edited by Clive Seale, 143–159. Malden, Mass.: Blackwell, 2004.

Defensive Medicine and Medical Malpractice. Office of Technology Assessment. Washington, D.C.: U.S. Congress, July 1994. http://biotech.law.lsu.edu/policy/9405.pdf.

Defleur, Melvin L. "Occupational Roles as Portrayed on Television." *Public Opinion Quarterly* 28, no. 1 (March 20, 1964): 57–74. doi:10.1086/267221.

DeNavas-Walt, Carmet, Bernadette D. Proctor, and Jessica D. Smith. *Income, Poverty, and Health Insurance Coverage in the United States: 2010.* Current Population Reports. Washington, D.C.: U.S. Department of Commerce, 2011.

Disease, Immunization and Respiratory. "CDC - SARS - Basics Fact Sheet." Accessed January 15, 2014. http://www.cdc.gov/sars/about/fs-SARS.html.

Eagleton, Terry. *Ideology: An Introduction.* New and Updated Edition edition. London; New York: Verso, 2007.

Ehrenreich, Barbara, and Deirdre English. *For Her Own Good: Two Centuries of the Experts' Advice to Women.* New York: Anchor Books, 2005.

Emanuel, E.J., and L.L. Emanuel. "Four Models of the Physician-Patient Relationship." *JAMA: The Journal of the American Medical Association* 267, no. 16 (April 22, 1992): 2221–2226.

Engel, Jonathan. *Poor People's Medicine: Medicaid and American Charity Care since 1965.* Durham, NC: Duke Univ. Press, 2006.

Enough Is Enough (No More Tears). Television program. Grey's Anatomy. ShondaLand, The Mark Gordon Company, Touchstone Television, & ABC Studios, 2005.

Epstein, R.M., Alper, B.S., and Quill, T.E. "Communicating Evidence for Participatory Decision Making." *JAMA* 291, no. 19 (May 19, 2004): 2359–2366. doi:10.1001/jama.291.19.2359.

"ER: On the Beach." TV.com. Accessed June 11, 2014. http://www.tv.com/shows/er/on-the-beach-130896/.

Faith. Television program. ER. Warner Brothers, 1997.

Family Matters. Television program. ER. Warner Brothers, 2000.

Fear of Flying. Television program. ER. Warner Brothers, 1996.

Feb. 5, '95. Television program. ER. Warner Brothers, 1995.

Fidelity. Television program. House, M.D. Bad Hat Harry Productions, 2004.

Flanagan-Klygis, E.A., Sharp, L., and Frader, J.E. "Dismissing the Family Who Refuses Vaccines: A Study of Pediatrician Attitudes." *Archives of Pediatrics & Adolescent Medicine* 159, no. 10 (October 1, 2005): 929–934. doi:10.1001/archpedi.159.10.929.

Food Chains of Chicago Hope. Television program. Chicago Hope. 20th Century Fox, 1994.

Fortune, Jennifer, and Kumanan Wilson. "Preserving Relationships with Antivaccine Parents: Five Suggestions from Social Psychology." *Canadian Family Physician* 53, no. 12 (December 1, 2007): 2083–2085.

Francis, Roberta W. "The History behind the Equal Rights Amendment." *The Equal Rights Amendment,* 2005. http://equalrightsamendment.org/history.htm.

Gauthier, Candace Cummins. "Television Drama and Popular Film as Medical Narrative." *Journal of American Culture* 22, no. 3 (1999): 23–25. doi:10.1111/j.1542-734X.1999.2203_23.x.

Gaynes, Robert. *Germ Theory: Medical Pioneers in Infectious Diseases.* 1st edition. Washington, DC: ASM Press, 2011.

Gerbner, George, and Larry Gross. "Living with Television: The Violence Profile." *Journal of Communication* 26, no. 2 (1976): 172–94. doi:10.1111/j.1460-2466.1976.tb01397.x.

Gerbner, George, Larry Gross, Michael Morgan, and Nancy Signmorielli. "Health and Medicine on Television." *The New England Journal of Medicine* 305, no. 15 (1981): 901–4.

Get Carter. Television program. ER. Warner Brothers, 2004.

Gibson, Rosemary, and Janardan Prasad Singh. *Wall of Silence: The Untold Story of the Medical Mistakes That Kill and Injure Millions of Americans.* Washington, D.C.; Lanham, MD: LifeLine Press ; Distributed to the trade by National Book Network, 2003.

Gitlin, Todd. "Prime Time Ideology: The Hegemonic Process in Television Entertainment." *Social Problems* 26, no. 3 (February 1979): 251–66. doi:10.2307/800451.

Glannon, Walter. "Responsibility, Alcoholism, and Liver Transplantation." *Journal of Medicine and Philosophy* 23, no. 1 (1998): 31–49. doi:10.1076/jmep.23.1.31.2595.

Glatter, Lesli Linka. *Let It Be.* Television program. Grey's Anatomy. ShondaLand, The Mark Gordon Company, Touchstone Television, & ABC Studios, 2005.

Glik, Deborah, Emil Berkanovic, Kathleen Stone, Leticia Ibarra, Marcy Connell Jones, Bob Rosen, Myrl Schreibman, Lisa Gordon, Laura Minassian, and Darcy Richardes. "Health Education Goes Hollywood: Working with Prime-Time and Daytime Entertainment Television for Immunization Promotion." *Journal of Health Communication* 3, no. 3 (1998): 263–282. doi:10.1080/108107398127364.

Ground Zero. Television program. ER. Warner Brothers, 1997.

Hall, Stuart. "The Rediscovery of 'Ideology': Return of the Repressed in Media Studies." In *Cultural Theory and Popular Culture: A Reader*, edited by John Storey, 3rd ed., 124–55. Pearson Prentice Hall, 2006.

Hall, Stuart, Jessica Evans, and Sean Nixon. *Representation: Cultural Representations and Signifying Practices.* Second Edition. Los Angeles : Milton Keynes, United Kingdom: SAGE Publications Ltd, 2013.

Haller, Beth A. *Representing Disability in an Ableist World: Essays on Mass Media.* Louisville, KY: The Advocado Press, 2010.

Hardey, Michael. "Doctor in the House: The Internet as a Source of Lay Health Knowledge and the Challenge to Expertise." *Sociology of Health & Illness* 21, no. 6 (1999): 820–835. doi:10.1111/1467-9566.00185.

Health, CDC's Office on Smoking and. "Smoking and Tobacco Use; Fact Sheet; Adult Cigarette Smoking in the United States;." *Smoking and Tobacco Use.* Accessed January 15, 2014. http://www.cdc.gov/tobacco/data_statistics/fact_sheets/adult_data/cig_smoking/.

Health, CDC's Office on Smoking and. "Smoking and Tobacco Use; Fact Sheet; Youth and Tobacco Use." *Smoking and Tobacco Use.* Accessed January 15, 2014. http://www.cdc.gov/tobacco/data_statistics/fact_sheets/youth_data/tobacco_use/.

Health, Education, and Welfare U. S. Department of. *Healthy People: The Surgeon General's Report on Health Promotion and Disease Prevention, 1979.* 1st edition. U.S. Department of Health, Education, and Welfare, n.d.

Healthy People 2000: National Health Promotion and Disease Objectives. U.S. Department of Health and Human Services, 1990.

Heath, Chip, and Heath, Dan. *Switch: How to Change Things When Change Is Hard.* London: Random House, 2011.

Heavy. Television program. House, M.D. Bad Hat Harry Productions, n.d.

HHS Announces $50 Million Investment to Patient Safety. 2001 Press Release Archive. Agency for Healthcare Research and Quality, October 11, 2001. http://archive.ahrq.gov/news/press/pr2001/patsafpr.htm.

Hilts, Philip J. *Protecting America's Health: The FDA, Business, and One Hundred Years of Regulation.* Chapel Hill: University of North Carolina Press, 2004.

Holcomb, Rod. *Last Call.* Television program. Warner Brothers, 1996.

Horwitz, Leora I., Jeremy Green, and Elizabeth H. Bradley. "US Emergency Department Performance on Wait Time and Length of Visit." *Annals of Emergency Medicine* 55, no. 2 (February 2010): 133–141. doi:10.1016/j.annemergmed.2009.07.023.

House of Cards. Television program. ER. Warner Brothers, 1995.

House Training. Television program. House, M.D. Bad Hat Harry Productions, 2007.

"How Authentic Is Medicine on Television?" *JAMA: The Journal of the American Medical Association* (May 1957): 49–51.

Hudson, Angela L., Adeline Nyamathi, Barbara Greengold, Alexandra Slagle, Deborah Koniak-Griffin, Farinaz Khalilifard, and Daniel Getzoff. "Health-Seeking Challenges Among Homeless Youth." *Nursing Research* 59, no. 3 (2010): 212–218. doi:10.1097/NNR.0b013e3181d1a8a9.

Humpty Dumpty. Television program. House, M.D. Bad Hat Harry Productions, 2005.

Iezzoni, Lisa I., Sowmya R. Rao, Catherine M. DesRoches, Christine Vogeli, and Eric G. Campbell. "Survey Shows That At Least Some Physicians Are Not Always Open Or Honest With Patients." *Health Affairs* 31, no. 2 (February 1, 2012): 383–391. doi:10.1377/hlthaff.2010.1137.

Increased Safety-Belt Use—United States, 1991. MMWR Weekly. Centers for Disease Control, June 19, 1992.

Insurrection. Television program. ER. Warner Brothers, 2002.

Into That Good Night. Television program. ER. Warner Brothers, 1994.

Irwin, Don. "Reagan Stresses Family Values While Hart Laments Iran Scandal." *Los Angeles Times*, December 21, 1986. http://articles.latimes.com/1986-12-21/news/mn-4286_1_gary-hart.

Iverson, Suzy A., Kristin B. Howard, and Brian K. Penney. "Impact of Internet Use on Health-Related Behaviors and the Patient-Physician Relationship: A Survey-Based Study and Review." *JAOA: Journal of the American Osteopathic Association* 108, no. 12 (December 1, 2008): 699–711.

Jacobs, Jason. *Body Trauma TV: The New Hospital Dramas*. London: British Film Institute, 2003.

Jaffe, Matthew, Kate Barrett, and Tom Shine. "Dennis Quaid Talks Medical Errors with Congress." *ABC News*, May 14, 2008. http://abcnews.go.com/Health/story?id=4848865&page=1.

Jensen, Klaus, and Nick Jankowski. *A Handbook of Qualitative Methodologies for Mass Communication Research*. London [etc.]: Routledge, 1991.

Jepson, R.G., L. Mihaljevic, and J. Craig. "Cranberries for Preventing Urinary Tract Infections." *The Cochrane Database of Systematic Reviews* no. 2 (2004): CD001321. doi:10.1002/14651858.CD001321.pub3.

Johnson, Steven. *The Ghost Map: The Story of London's Most Terrifying Epidemic—and How It Changed Science, Cities, and the Modern World*. Penguin, 2006.

Jones, Elka. "As Seen on TV: Reality vs. Fantasy in Occupational Portrayals on the Small Screen. Watch Television for Clues about Working, and You Might Be Entertained. But Watch TV to Make Career Decisions, and You Might Not Be Ready for Prime Time." *Occupational Outlook Quarterly*, 2003. Academic OneFile.

Jones, Mark. *ER: The Unofficial Guide*. London: Contender, 2003.

Kalisch, Philip A., and Beatrice J. Kalisch. "A Comparative Analysis of Nurse and Physician Characters in the Entertainment Media." *Journal of Advanced Nursing* 11, no. 2 (1986): 179–195. doi:10.1111/j.1365-2648.1986.tb01236.x.

Kaplan, Jonathan. *A Shot in the Dark*. Television program. ER. Warner Brothers, 2004.

———. *Orion in the Sky*. Television program. ER. Warner Brothers, 2002.

Karmen, Andrew. *Crime Victims: An Intro to Victimology*. [s.l.]: Wadsworth, 2012.

Kelley, David E. *Broken Hearts*. Television program. Chicago Hope. 20th Century Fox, 1998.

Kirkwood, William G., and Dan Brown. "Public Communication About the Causes of Disease: The Rhetoric of Responsibility." *Journal of Communication* 45, no. 1 (1995): 55–76. doi:10.1111/j.1460-2466.1995.tb00714.x.

Kletke, Phillip R., William D. Marder, Anne B. Silberger, and Center for Health Policy Research (American Medical Association). *The Demographics of Physician Supply: Trends and Projections*. Chicago, IL: American Medical Association, 1987.

Kubiak, Sheryl Pimlott, Kristine Siefert, and Carol J. Boyd. "Empowerment and Public Policy: An Exploration of the Implications of Section 115 of the Personal Responsibility and Work Opportunity Act." *Journal of Community Psychology* 32, no. 2 (2004): 127–143. doi:10.1002/jcop.10088.

Kushel, M.B., Vittinghoff, E., and Haas, J.S. "Factors Associated with the HealthCare Utilization of Homeless Persons." *JAMA* 285, no. 2 (January 10, 2001): 200–206. doi:10.1001/jama.285.2.200.

Kushel, Margot B., Sharon Perry, David Bangsberg, Richard Clark, and Andrew R. Moss. "Emergency Department Use Among the Homeless and Marginally Housed: Results from a Community-Based Study." *American Journal of Public Health* 92, no. 5 (May 2002): 778–784. doi:10.2105/AJPH.92.5.778.

Laham, Nicholas. *A Lost Cause: Bill Clinton's Campaign for National Health Insurance*. Westport, Conn.: Praeger, 1996.

Lamb to the Slaughter. Television program. Chicago Hope. 20th Century Fox, 1997.

Larsen, Peter. "Textual Analysis of Fictional Media Content." In *A Handbook of Qualitative Methodologies for Mass Communication Research*, 121–34. London: Routledge, 1991.

Le Fanu, James. *The Rise and Fall of Modern Medicine*. New York: Basic Books, 2012.

Leask, Julie, Paul Kinnersley, Cath Jackson, Francine Cheater, Helen Bedford, and Greg Rowles. "Communicating with Parents about Vaccination: A Framework for Health Professionals." *BMC Pediatrics* 12, no. 1 (December 1, 2012): 1–11. doi:10.1186/1471-2431-12-154.

Leggo My Ego. Television program. Chicago Hope. 20th Century Fox, n.d.

Levy, A.S., and R.C. Stokes. "Effects of a Health Promotion Advertising Campaign on Sales of Ready-to-Eat Cereals." *Public Health Reports* 102, no. 4 (1987): 398–403.

Lewis, Richard. *Pirates of the Third Reich*. Television program. C.S.I. Crime Scene Investigation. Alliance Atlantis Communications, 2006.

Loose Ends. Television program. ER. Warner Brothers, 2000.

MacDonald, J.F. "Black Doctors on Television." *New York State Journal of Medicine* 85, no. 4 (April 1985): 151–152.

Makoul, Gregory, and Limor Peer. "Dissecting the Doctor Shows: A Content Analysis of ER and Chicago Hope." In *Cultural Sutures: Medicine and Media*, edited by Lester D. Friedman, 244–262. Durham, N.C.: Duke University Press, 2004.

Mann, Seith. *Don't Stand So Close to Me*. Television program. ER. ShondaLand, The Mark Gordon Company, Touchstone Television, & ABC Studios, 2006.

Marmor, Theodore R. *Understanding Health Care Reform*, New Haven: Yale University Press, 1994.

Martins, Diane Cocozza. "Experiences of Homeless People in the Health Care Delivery System: A Descriptive Phenomenological Study." *Public Health Nursing* 25, no. 5 (2008): 420–430. doi:10.1111/j.1525-1446.2008.00726.x.

Marvel, M., Epstein, R.M., Flowers, K., and Beckman, H.B. "Soliciting the Patient's Agenda: Have We Improved?" *JAMA* 281, no. 3 (January 20, 1999): 283–287. doi:10.1001/jama.281.3.283.

McLaughlin, James. "The Doctor Shows." *Journal of Communication* 25, no. 3 (1975): 182–84. doi:10.1111/j.1460-2466.1975.tb00623.x.

Meaning. Television program. House, M.D. Bad Hat Harry Productions, 2006.

Metzl, Jonathan Michel. *Prozac on the Couch: Prescribing Gender in the Era of Wonder Drugs*. Durham: Duke University Press Books, 2003.

Millenson, Michael L. "The Silence." *Health Affairs* 22, no. 2 (March 1, 2003): 103–112. doi:10.1377/hlthaff.22.2.103.

Mindich, David T. Z. *Just the Facts: How Objectivity Came to Define American Journalism*. NYU Press, 2000.

Minkler, Meredith. "Personal Responsibility for Health? A Review of the Arguments and the Evidence at Century's End." *Health Education & Behavior* 26, no. 1 (February 1, 1999): 121–141. doi:10.1177/109019819902600110.

Misiano, Christopher. *Great Expectations*. ER. Warner Brothers, 1999.

Missing. Television program. ER. Warner Brothers, 2003.

"Mission and Vision | National Patient Safety Foundation." Accessed January 15, 2014. http://www.npsf.org/about-us/mission-and-vision/.

Moore, Tom. *Let the Games Begin*. Television program. ER. Warner Brothers, 1996.

Morgan, Susan E., Tyler R. Harrison, Walid A. Afifi, Shawn D. Long, and Michael T. Stephenson. "In Their Own Words: The Reasons Why People Will (Not) Sign an Organ Donor Card." *Health Communication* 23, no. 1 (2008): 23–33. doi:10.1080/10410230701805158.

Morrow, M., Jagsi, R., Alderman, A.K., and et al. "Surgeon Recommendations and Receipt of Mastectomy for Treatment of Breast Cancer." *JAMA* 302, no. 14 (October 14, 2009): 1551–1556. doi:10.1001/jama.2009.1450.

"Multiple Sclerosis." Text. Accessed January 15, 2014. http://www.nlm.nih.gov/medlineplus/multiplesclerosis.html.

Murray, E., Lo, B., Pollack, L., and et al. "The Impact of Health Information on the Internet on the Physician-Patient Relationship: Patient Perceptions." *Archives of Internal Medicine* 163, no. 14 (July 28, 2003): 1727–1734. doi:10.1001/archinte.163.14.1727.

Muzio, Gloria. *I Do*. Television program. ER. Warner Brothers, 2005.

———. *Refusal of Care*. Television program. ER. Warner Brothers, 2005.

———. *TB or Not TB*. Television program. House, M.D. Bad Hat Harry Productions, 2005.

National Institutes of Health. *Opportunities and Challenges in Digestive Diseases Research: Recommendations of the National Commission on Digestive Diseases.* Bethesda, MD: U.S. Department of Health and Human Services, n.d.

No Good Deed Goes Unpunished. Television program. ER. Warner Brothers, 2003.

Nordenberg, Tamar. "Make no mistake! Medical errors can be deadly serious." *FDA consumer* 34, no. 5 (1999): 13–18.

Norris, Pippa. "Skeptical Patients: Performance, Social Capital, and Culture." In *The Trust Crisis in Healthcare,* edited by David A. Shore, 32–48. Oxford; New York: Oxford University Press, 2007.

Nurit, Guttman, and William Harris Ressler. "On Being Responsible: Ethical Issues in Appeals to Personal Responsibility in Health Campaigns." *Journal of Health Communication* 6, no. 2 (2001): 117–136. doi:10.1080/10810730116864.

O'Connor, M.M. "The Role of the Television Drama ER in Medical Student Life: Entertainment or Socialization?" *JAMA: The Journal of the American Medical Association* 280, no. 9 (September 2, 1998): 854–55.

O'Fallon, Peter. *Paternity.* Television program. House, M.D. Bad Hat Harry Productions, 2004.

"Obesity and Overweight for Professionals: Childhood: Data | DNPAO | CDC." Accessed January 15, 2014. http://www.cdc.gov/obesity/data/childhood.html.

Occam's Razor. Television program. House, M.D. Bad Hat Harry Productions, 2004.

Office of Communications and Public Liaison. "Spinal Cord Injury: Hope Through Research." *National Institute of Neurological Disorders and Stroke,* July 1, 2013. http://www.ninds.nih.gov/disorders/sci/detail_sci.htm#Organizations.

Ogden, Cynthia L., Margaret D. Carroll, Brian K. Kit, and Katherine M. Flegal. "Prevalence of Obesity in the United States, 2009–2010." *NCHS Data Brief* no. 82 (January 2012): 1–8.

Oh, the Guilt. Television program. Grey's Anatomy. ShondaLand, The Mark Gordon Company, Touchstone Television, & ABC Studios, 2006.

Omer, S.B., Pan, W.Y., Halsey, N.A., et al. "Nonmedical Exemptions to School Immunization Requirements: Secular Trends and Association of State Policies with Pertussis Incidence." *JAMA* 296, no. 14 (October 11, 2006): 1757–1763. doi:10.1001/jama.296.14.1757.

"Organdonor.gov | The Need Is Real: Data." Html, May 25, 2011. http://organdonor.gov/about/data.html.

Østbye, Truls, Bill Miller, and Heather Keller. "Throw That Epidemiologist out of the Emergency Room! Using the Television Series ER as a Vehicle for Teaching Methodologists about Medical Issues." *Journal of Clinical Epidemiology* 50, no. 10 (October 1997): 1183–86. doi:10.1016/S0895-4356(97)00178-9.

Parrott, Roxanne. "Advocate or Adversary?: The Self-reflexive Roles of Media Messages for Health." *Critical Studies in Mass Communication* 13, no. 3 (1996): 266–78. doi:10.1080/15295039609366979.

"Patients Doubt Doctors' Advice When It Conflicts With Online Info - iHealthBeat." Accessed January 15, 2014. http://www.ihealthbeat.org/articles/2008/7/30/patients-doubt-doctors-advice-when-it-conflicts-with-online-info.

Pe, Fine. "Herd Immunity: History, Theory, Practice." *Epidemiologic Reviews* 15, no. 2 (December 1992): 265–302.

Peruzzi, Alfred. "View Askew. What Is Degrading the Teaching Hospital's Image?" *Marketing Health Services* 26, no. 2 (2006): 44.

Peterson, Michael W., and Peter C. Fretz. "Patient Use of the Internet for Information in a Lung Cancer Clinic." *CHEST Journal* 123, no. 2 (February 1, 2003): 452–457. doi:10.1378/chest.123.2.452.

Pfau, Michael, Lawrence J. Mullen, and Kirsten Garrow. "The Influence of Television Viewing on Public Perceptions of Physicians." *Journal of Broadcasting & Electronic Media* 39, no. 4 (1995): 441–458. doi:10.1080/08838159509364318.

Pham, Julius Cuong, Monica S. Aswani, Michael Rosen, HeeWon Lee, Matthew Huddle, Kristina Weeks, and Peter J. Pronovost. "Reducing Medical Errors and Adverse Events." *Annual Review of Medicine* 63, no. 1 (2012): 447–463. doi:10.1146/annurev-med-061410-121352.

Platt, David. *Starved*. Television program. Law & Order: Special Victims United. Wolf Films, 2005.

Post Mortem. Television program. ER. Warner Brothers, 1997.

Raben, Estelle Manette. "Men in White and Yellow Jack as Mirrors of the Medical Profession." *Literature and Medicine* 12, no. 1 (1993): 19–41. doi:10.1353/lm.2011.0235.

Reducing Tobacco Use: A Report of the Surgeon General. MMWR: Recommendations and Reports. Centers for Disease Control, December 22, 2000. http://www.cdc.gov/mmwr/preview/mmwrhtml/rr4916a1.htm.

Reeves, Jimmie L., Richard Campbell, and Richard Cambell. *Cracked Coverage: Television News, The Anti-Cocaine Crusade, and the Reagan Legacy*. Duke University Press, 2012.

Reger, B., M.G. Wootan, S. Booth-Butterfield, and H. Smith. "1% or Less: A Community-Based Nutrition Campaign." *Public Health Reports* 113, no. 5 (1998): 410–419.

Research, Center for Drug Evaluation and. "Information for Consumers (Drugs) - Strategies to Reduce Medication Errors: Working to Improve Medication Safety." WebContent. Accessed January 15, 2014. http://www.fda.gov/Drugs/ResourcesForYou/Consumers/ucm143553.htm.

Rimes, Shonda. *The Self-Destruct Button*. Television program. Grey's Anatomy. ShondaLand, The Mark Gordon Company, Touchstone Television, and ABC Studios, 2005.

Rimes, Shonda. *Shake Your Groove Thing*. Television program. Grey's Anatomy. Shonda-Land, The Mark Gordon Company, Touchstone Television, & ABC Studios, 2005.

Robinson, Jule Anne. *Band Aid Covers the Bullet Hole*. Television program. Grey's Anatomy. ShondaLand, The Mark Gordon Company, Touchstone Television, & ABC Studios, 2006.

Rothman, Ellen L., and Ellen *White Coat: Becoming a Doctor at Harvard Medical School*. 1st edition. New York, NY. William Morrow Paperbacks, 2000.

Safran, Dana Gelb. "Patients' Trust in Their Doctors: Are We Losing Ground?" In *The Trust Crisis in Healthcare*, edited by David A Shore, 79–88. Oxford; New York: Oxford University Press, 2007.

Samji, Hasina, Angela Cescon, Robert S. Hogg, Sharada P. Modur, Keri N. Althoff, Kate Buchacz, Ann N. Burchell, et al. "Closing the Gap: Increases in Life Expectancy among Treated HIV-Positive Individuals in the United States and Canada." *PLoS ONE* 8, no. 12 (December 18, 2013): e81355. doi:10.1371/journal.pone.0081355.

Sandman, Peter M. "Medicine and Mass Communication: An Agenda for Physicians." *Annals of Internal Medicine* 85, no. 3 (September 1, 1976): 378–83. doi:10.7326/0003-4819-85-3-378.

Sarafian, Deran. *Autopsy*. Television program. House, M.D. Bad Hat Harry Productions, 2005.

Schulman, Bruce J. *The Seventies: The Great Shift in American Culture, Society, and Politics*. Cambridge, Mass.: Da Capo, 2002.

Scott, Oz. *Genevieve and the Fat Boy*. Television program. Chicago Hope. 20th Century Fox, 1994.

Shale, Richard. "Images of the Medical Pofession in the Movies." *Ohio State Medical Journal* 80, no. 11 (1984): 775–79.

"Second Opinions: Greater Understanding." *Patient Advocate Foundation*, 2012. http://www.patientadvocate.org/index.php?p=691.

"Second Surgical Opinions." *Medicare.gov: The Official U.S. Government Site for Medicare*. Accessed January 15, 2014. http://www.medicare.gov/coverage/second-surgical-opinions.html.

Sharf, Barbara F., and Vicki S. Freimuth. "The Construction of Illness on Entertainment Television: Coping with Cancer on Thirtysomething." *Health Communication* 5, no. 3 (1993): 141–160. doi:10.1207/s15327027hc0503_1.

Shen, Joannie, Ronald Andersen, Paul S. Albert, Neil Wenger, John Glaspy, Melissa Cole, and Paul Shekelle. "Use of Complementary/Alternative Therapies by Women with Advanced-Stage Breast Cancer." *BMC Complementary and Alternative Medicine* 2, no. 1 (August 13, 2002): 8. doi:10.1186/1472-6882-2-8.

Shifts Happen. Television program. ER. Warner Brothers, 2003.

Shore, David A. *Daddy's Boy*. Television program. House, M.D. Bad Hat Harry Productions, 2005.

————. *Que Será Será.* Television program. House, M.D. Bad Hat Harry Productions, 2006.

————. *The Mistake.* Television program. House, M.D. Bad Hat Harry Productions, 2005.

————. *The Trust Crisis in Healthcare: Causes, Consequences, and Cures.* Oxford; New York: Oxford University Press, 2007.

Siegel, Rebecca, Jiemin Ma, Zhaohui Zou, and Ahmedin Jemal. "Cancer Statistics, 2014." *CA: A Cancer Journal for Clinicians* (2014): n/a–n/a. doi:10.3322/caac.21208.

Singhal, Arvind. *Entertainment-Education and Social Change: History, Research, and Practice.* Mahwah, N.J.: Lawrence Erlbaum Associates, 2004.

Singer, Bryan. *Pilot.* Television program. House, M.D. Bad Hat Harry Productions, 2004.

"Smoking Bans Cut Number of Heart Attacks, Strokes." Accessed January 15, 2014. http://www.usatoday.com/story/news/nation/2012/10/29/smoking-bans-heart-attacks-strokes/1664193/.

Soumerai, Stephen B., Dennis Ross-Degnan, and Jessica Spira Kahn. "The Effects of Professional and Media Warnings About the Association Between Aspirin Use in Children and Reye's Syndrome." In *Public Health Communication: Evidence for Behavior Change*, edited by Robert Hornik. Mahwah, N.J.: Taylor & Francis, 2008.

Spath, Patrice. *Error Reduction in Health Care: A Systems Approach to Improving Patient Safety.* San Francisco, Calif.: Jossey-Bass, 2011.

Staff, Pew Research Center's Journalism Project. "What Americans Learned From the Media About the Health Care Debate." *Pew Research Center's Journalism Project*, June 19, 2012.

Starr, Paul. *Remedy and Reaction: The Peculiar American Struggle over Health Care Reform.* New Haven: Yale University Press, 2013.

Starr, Paul. *The Social Transformation of American Medicine.* New York: Basic Books, 1982.

Steinbrook, Robert. "Imposing Personal Responsibility for Health." *New England Journal of Medicine* 355, no. 8 (2006): 753–756. doi:10.1056/NEJMp068141.

"STD Trends in the United States, 2010." Accessed January 15, 2014. http://www.cdc.gov/std/stats10/trends.htm.

Street, 1615 L., NW, Suite 700 Washington, and DC 20036 202 419 4300 | Main 202 419 4349 | Fax 202 419 4372 | Media Inquiries. "Key News Audiences Now Blend Online and Traditional Sources." *Pew Research Center for the People and the Press*, August 17, 2008. http://www.people-press.org/2008/08/17/key-news-audiences-now-blend-online-and-traditional-sources/.

————. "Public Remains Split on Health Care Bill, Opposed to Mandate." *Pew Research Center for the People and the Press*, March 26, 2012. http://www.people-press.org/2012/03/26/public-remains-split-on-health-care-bill-opposed-to-mandate/.

Studdert, D.M., Mello, M.M., Sage, W.M., and et al. "Defensive Medicine among High-Risk Specialist Physicians in a Volatile Malpractice Environment." *JAMA* 293, no. 21 (June 1, 2005): 2609–2617. doi:10.1001/jama.293.21.2609.

Such Sweet Sorrow. Television program. ER. Warner Brothers, 2000.

Sugerman, David E., Albert E. Barskey, Maryann G. Delea, Ismael R. Ortega-Sanchez, Daoling Bi, Kimberly J. Ralston, Paul A. Rota, Karen Waters-Montijo, and Charles W. LeBaron. "Measles Outbreak in a Highly Vaccinated Population, San Diego, 2008: Role of the Intentionally Undervaccinated." *Pediatrics* 125, no. 4 (April 1, 2010): 747–755. doi:10.1542/peds.2009-1653.

Summers, Sandy Jacobs, and Harry Jacobs Summers. "Viewpoint: Media 'Nursing': Retiring the Handmaiden." *The American Journal of Nursing* 104, no. 2 (February 1, 2004): 13.

"Super Bowl 2010 Ratings: 106 Million Watch, Top-Rated Telecast EVER." *Huffington Post.* Accessed June 14, 2014. http://www.huffingtonpost.com/2010/02/08/super-bowl-2010-ratings-m_n_453503.html.

"Surgical Implements Too Often Left Behind in Patients: Report." *Health News / Tips & Trends / Celebrity Health.* Accessed January 15, 2014. http://news.health.com/2013/10/17/surgical-implements-too-often-left-behind-in-patients-report/.

"Tarnished Images, Plus a Few Gems." *Nursing* 38, no. 3 (March 2008): 28–29. doi:10.1097/01.NURSE.0000312617.59187.e8.

"Television as a Health Educator: A Case Study of Grey's Anatomy." Accessed January 16, 2014. http://kff.org/other/television-as-a-health-educator-a-case/.

"Television as a Health Educator: A Case Study of Grey's Anatomy." Accessed June 6, 2014. http://kff.org/other/television-as-a-health-educator-a-case/.

Tell Me Sweet Little Lies. Television program. Grey's Anatomy, 2006.

Teng, Larry. *God Complex.* Television program. Criminal Minds. Mark Gordon Company, 2012.

Tesh, Sylvia Noble. *Hidden Arguments: Political Ideology and Disease Prevention Policy.* New Brunswick, N.J.: Rutgers University Press, 1988.

The Crossing. Television program. ER. Warner Brothers, 2001.

The Deficit Reduction Act: Important Facts for State Government Officials. Department of Health and Human Services. Accessed January 14, 2014. http://www.cms.gov/Regulations-and- Guidance/Legislation/DeficitReductionAct/downloads/Checklist1.pdf.

The Ethics of Hope. Television program. Chicago Hope. 20th Century Fox, 1995.

The Providers. Television program. ER. Warner Brothers, 2005.

The Self-Destruct Button. Television program. Grey's Anatomy. ShondaLand, The Mark Gordon Company, Touchstone Television, & ABC Studios, 2005.

The Visit. Television program. ER. Warner Brothers, 2000.

Think Warm Thoughts. Television program. ER. Warner Brothers, 1998.

Three Stories. Television program. House, M.D. Warner Brothers, 2005.

"Trends in In-Hospital Newborn Male Circumcision — United States, 1999–2010." Accessed January 16, 2014. http://www.cdc.gov/mmwr/preview/mmwrhtml/mm6034a4.htm.

Trevino, Jesus Salvador. *Second Chances.* Television program. Chicago Hope. 20th Century Fox, 1996.

Tribes. Television program. ER. Warner Brothers, 1997.

Tu, Ha, T., and Genna R. Cohen. "Striking Jump in Consumers Seeking Health Care Information." *Tracking Report / Center for Studying Health System Change* no. 20 (August 2008): 1–8.

Turow, J. "Television Entertainment and the US Health-Care Debate." *The Lancet* 347, no. 9010 (May 1996): 1240–1243. doi:10.1016/S0140-6736(96)90747-3.

Turow, Joseph. *Playing Doctor: Television, Storytelling, and Medical Power.* The University of Michigan Press, 2010.

Under Control. ER. Warner Brothers, 2000.

"Updated Thursday Ratings: ER Finale Draws 16.2 Million Viewers." *TVbytheNumbers.* Accessed June 12, 2014. http://tvbythenumbers.zap2it.com/2009/04/03/thursday-ratings-er-draws-163-million-viewers/15864/.

Uppendahl, Michael. *Nor'easter.* Television program. American Horror Story. Brad Falchuk Teley-Vision, Ryan Murphy Productions, 20th Century Fox, 2012.

Vandekieft, Gregg. "From City Hospital to ER: The Evolution of the Television Physician." In *Cultural Sutures: Medicine and Media,* 215–33. Durham, N.C.: Duke University Press, 2004.

Vanishing Act. Television program. Warner Brothers, 1998.

Volgy, Thomas J., and John E. Schwarz. "TV Entertainment Programming and Sociopolitical Attitudes." *Journalism Quarterly* 57, no. 1 (January 1980): 150–55.

Wachter, Robert M., and Kaveh G. Shojania. *Internal Bleeding: The Truth behind America's Terrifying Epidemic of Medical Mistakes.* New York City: Rugged Land, 2005.

Wells, John. "On the Beach." ER. NBC, May 9, 2002.

Wang, Caroline. "Culture, Meaning and Disability: Injury Prevention Campaigns and the Production of Stigma." *Social Science & Medicine* 35, no. 9 (November 1992): 1093–1102. doi:10.1016/0277-9536(92)90221-B.

"We Look Back At The Top TV Shows of 2002." *TVbytheNumbers.* Accessed June 11, 2014. http://tvbythenumbers.zap2it.com/2008/04/26/we-look-back-at-the-top-tv-shows-of-2002/3513/.

Wells, John. *A Walk in the Woods.* Television program. ER. Warner Brothers, 2001.

Whang, Gilbert, Greg T. Mogel, Jerome Tsai, and Suzanne L. Palmer. "Left Behind: Unintentionally Retained Surgically Placed Foreign Bodies and How to Reduce Their Incidence—Pictorial Review." *American Journal of Roentgenology* 193, no. 6 supplement (December 2009): S79–S89. doi:10.2214/AJR.09.7153.

When the Bough Breaks. Television program. ER. Warner Brothers, 1997.

White, Dean. *Silencer*. Television program. Law & Order: Special Victims United. Wolf Films, 2007.

Who's Zoomin' Who? Television program. Grey's Anatomy. ShondaLand, The Mark Gordon Company, Touchstone Television, & ABC Studios, 2005.

Williams, Raymond. *Culture and Society 1780–1950*. 2nd edition. New York: Columbia University Press, 1983.

Wilson, Fernando A., and Jim P. Stimpson. "Trends in Fatalities from Distracted Driving in the United States, 1999 to 2008." *American Journal of Public Health* 100, no. 11 (November 2010): 2213–2219. doi:10.2105/AJPH.2009.187179.

Winsten, J.A. "Promoting Designated Drivers: The Harvard Alcohol Project." *American Journal of Preventive Medicine* 10, no. 3 Suppl (June 1994): 11–14.

Wuthnow, Robert. *American Mythos: Why Our Best Efforts to Be a Better Nation Fall Short*. Princeton: Princeton University Press, 2006.

You Bet Your Life. Television program. ER. Warner Brothers, 1997.

Zelman, Walter A. *The Changing Health Care Marketplace: Private Ventures, Public Interests*. San Francisco: Jossey-Bass Publishers, 1996.

Index

Index

CPSIA information can be obtained at www.ICGtesting.com
Printed in the USA
BVOW04*0507081014
369739BV00004B/5/P